A Guide to

Infection Control
in the Hospital

An official publication of the International Society for Infectious Diseases

R. Wenzel
USA

M. Edmond
USA

D. Pittet
Switzerland

J-M. Devaster
Belgium

T. Brewer
USA

A. Geddes
United Kingdom

J-P. Butzler
Belgium

1998
B.C. Decker Inc.
Hamilton • London

B.C. Decker Inc.
4 Hughson Street South
P.O. Box 620, L.C.D. 1
Hamilton, Ontario L8N 3K7
Tel: 905-522-7017; Fax: 905-522-7839
e-mail: info@bcdecker.com
Website: http//www.bcdecker.com

98 99 00 01 / PC / 9 8 7 6 5 4 3 2 1
ISBN 1-55009-059-3

Sales and Distribution

United States
Blackwell Science Inc.
Commerce Place
350 Main Street
Malden, MA 02148
U.S.A.
Tel: 1-800-215-1000

Canada
B.C. Decker Inc.
4 Hughson Street South
P.O. Box 620, L.C.D. 1
Hamilton, Ontario L8N 3K7
Tel: 905-522-7017
Fax: 905-522-7839
e-mail: info@bcdecker.com
Website: http//www.bcdecker.com

Japan
Igaku-Shoin Ltd.
Foreign Publications Department
3-24-17 Hongo, Bunkyo-ku
Tokyo 113-8719, Japan
Tel: 3 3817 5680
Fax: 3 3815 7805
e-mail: tmbook@ba2.so-net.or.jp

U.K., Europe, Scandinavia, Middle East
Blackwell Science Ltd.
c/o Marston Book Services Ltd.
P.O. Box 87
Oxford OX2 0DT
England
Tel: 44-1865-79115

Australia
Blackwell Science Pty, Ltd.
54 University Street
Carlton, Victoria 3053
Australia
Tel: 03 9347 0300
Fax: 03 9349 3016

India
**Jaypee Brothers Medical Publishers
(Pvt) Ltd.**
B-3, Emsa House, 23/23B, Ansari Road
Daryagnj, P.B. 7193
New Delhi – 110002, India
Tel: 11-3272143
Fax: 11-3276490

Notice: The authors and publisher have made every effort to ensure that the patient
care recommended herein, including choice of drugs and drug dosages, is in accord
with the accepted standard and practice at the time of publication. However, since
research and regulation constantly change clinical standards, the reader is urged to
check recent publications and the product information sheet included in the package of each drug, which includes recommended doses, warnings, and contraindica-
tions. This is particularly important with new or infrequently used drugs.

EDITORS

Richard P. Wenzel, MD, MSc
Department of Internal Medicine
Medical College of Virginia
Virginia Commonwealth University
Richmond, Virginia

Michael Edmond, MD, MPH
Medical College of Virginia Hospitals
Virginia Commonwealth University
Richmond, Virginia

Didier Pittet, MD, MS
Infection Control Program
University Hospitals
Geneva, Switzerland

Jeanne-Marie Devaster, MD
University Hospitals St. Pierre,
    Brugmann, and Queen Fabiola
Brussels, Belgium

Timothy F. Brewer, MD, MPH
Brigham & Women's Hospital
Boston, Massachusetts

Alasdair Geddes, MD
University of Birmingham
    School of Medicine
Birmingham, UK

Jean-Paul Butzler, MD, PhD
University Hospitals St. Pierre,
    Brugmann, and Queen Fabiola
Brussels, Belgium

CONTRIBUTORS

Bruno Baršić, MD
Department of Infectious Diseases
University Hospital
Zagreb, Republic of Croatia

Werner E. Bischoff, MD
Division of Quality Health Care
Department of Internal Medicine
Medical College of Virginia Hospitals
Virginia Commonwealth University
Richmond, Virginia

Timothy F. Brewer, MD, MPH
Brigham & Women's Hospital
Boston, Massachusetts

Jean-Paul Butzler, MD, PhD
University Hospitals,
    Brugmann, and Queen Fabiola
Brussels, Belgium

Anne Dediste, MD
University Hospitals St Pierre,
    Brugmann, and Queen Fabiola
Brussels, Belgium

Jeanne-Marie Devaster, MD
University Hospitals St Pierre,
    Brugmann, and Queen Fabiola
Brussels, Belgium

Bradley N. Doebbeling, MD, MS
University of Iowa, Department of
    Internal Medicine
Iowa City, Iowa

Herbert L. DuPont, MD
University of Texas Health Sciences
    Center
St. Luke's Episcopal Hospital
Houston, Texas

Michael Edmond, MD, MPH
Medical College of Virginia Hospitals
Virginia Commonwealth University
Richmond, Virginia

Gerd Fätkenheuer, MD
Department of Internal Medicine
University Hospital, Cologne
Germany

Diane Franchi, MD
Department of Internal Medicine
Medical College of Virginia
Virginia Commonwealth University
Richmond, Virginia

Helen Giamarellou, MD
Laiko General Hospital
Ist Department, Proped. Medicine
Athens, Greece

Stephan Harbarth, MD
Infection Control Program
University Hospitals
Geneva, Switzerland

T.D. Healing, MSc, PhD
MERLIN
London, UK

P. Hoffman, BSc
Laboratory of Hospital Infection
Central Public Health Laboratory
London, UK

Günter Kampf, MD
Institute for Hygiene
Free University
Berlin, Germany

J.A.J.W. Kluytmans, MD, PhD
Ignatius Hospital Breda
Department of Clinical
  Microbiology
Breda, The Netherlands

Philippe Lepage, MD, PhD
Department of Pediatrics
Ambroise Paré Hospital
Mons, Belgium

Jack Levy, MD, PhD
Department of Pediatrics
St. Pierre University Hospital
Brussels, Belgium

Patience Mandisodza, MSc
University Hospitals St Pierre,
  Brugmann, and Queen Fabiola
Brussels, Belgium

Shaheen Mehtar, MBBS, FRCP
Public Health Department
South Cape/Karoo, Western Cape
Republic of South Africa

Mary D. Nettleman, MD, MS
Department of Internal Medicine
Medical College of Virginia
Virginia Commonwealth University
Richmond, Virginia

Johannes Oosterom, DVM, PhD
Department of Household and
  Consumer Studies
Wageningen Agricultural University
The Netherlands

Meena H. Patel, MD
Department of Internal Medicine
Medical College of Virginia
Virginia Commonwealth University
Richmond, Virginia

Didier Pittet, MD, MS
Infection Control Program
University Hospitals
Geneva, Switzerland

Samuel Ponce de Leon R., MD, MSc
Division of Hospital Epidemiology
  and Quality Care
Instituto nacional de la Nutricion
  "Salvador Zubiran"
Mexico City, Mexico

M. Sigfrido Rangel-Frausto, MD, MSc
Hospital Epidemiology Research Unit
National Medical Center
Mexican Institute for Social Security
Mexico

Marie-Claude Roy, MD, MSc
Department of Microbiology
Hôpital de l'Enfant-Jesus
Quebec City, Quebec, Canada

Slavko Schönwald, MD, PhD
Department of Infectious Diseases
University Hospital
Zagreb, Republic of Croatia

Harald Seifert, MD
Institute for Medical Microbiology
  and Hygiene
University of Cologne, Germany

Marc J. Struelens, MD, PhD
Department of Microbiology
Erasme University Hospital
Brussels, Belgium

Made Sutjita, MD
University of Texas Health Sciences
  Center
St. Luke's Episcopal Hospital
Houston, Texas

C.M.A. Swanink, MD, PhD
Department of Medical Microbiology
University Hospital St. Radboud
Nijmegen, Netherlands

Antoni Trilla, MD, MSc
Epidemiology and Health Services
    Research Unit
Hospital Clinic, University of
    Barcelona
Barcelona, Spain

Sheik Jalal Uddin, MSc
University Hospital St Pierre
Brussels, Belgium

Olivier Vandenberg, MD
University Hospitals St Pierre
Brussels, Belgium

Philippe Van de Perre, MD, PhD
Centre Muraz, Bobo Dioulasso
Burkina Faso

Paul E. Verweij, MD, PhD
Department of Medical Microbiology
University Hospital St. Radboud
Nijmegen, Netherlands

Margreet C. Vos, MD, PhD
Department of Microbiology and
    Infectious Diseases
Erasmus University Medical Center
Rotterdam, Netherlands

Andreas Voss, MD, PhD
Department of Medical Microbiology
University Hospital St. Radboud
Nijmegen, Netherlands

Constanze Wendt, MD, MS
Institute for Hygiene, Free University
Berlin, Germany

Richard P. Wenzel, MD, MSc
Department of Internal Medicine
Medical College of Virginia
Virginia Commonwealth University
Richmond, Virginia

Sergio B. Wey, MD, PhD
Infectious Diseases Division
Sao Paulo Federal Medical School
Sao Paulo, Brazil

Alice H.M. Wong, MD
Department of Internal Medicine
Medical College of Virginia
Virginia Commonwealth University
Richmond, Virginia

Michael T. Wong, NM, MD
Department of Internal Medicine
Medical College of Virginia
Virginia Commonwealth University
Richmond, Virginia

SEJ Young, FRCP
Private Practice
London, UK

INTRODUCTION

In developed countries, from 5 to 10% of patients admitted to acute care hospitals acquire an infection which was not present or incubating on admission. The attack rate for developing countries can exceed 25%. Such hospital-acquired, or nosocomial, infections add to the morbidity, mortality, and costs expected from the patients' underlying diseases alone.

Because of the illnesses, deaths, and added costs related to nosocomial infections, the field of infection control has grown in importance over the last 30 years. Although estimates vary regarding the proportion of nosocomial infections which are preventable, it may be as high as 20% in developed countries and as high as 40% or more in developing countries. Furthermore, in developed countries 5 to 10% of infections acquired in the hospital occur as part of an epidemic or cluster. The figure is larger for developing countries. The major point, however, is that all epidemics or clusters are preventable, and the opportunities are excellent for limiting the occurrence of such infections. What is required is attention to the basic principles of good infection control.

The booklet contains the principles designed to reduce the rate of nosocomial infections. They are intended to improve quality of care, minimize risk, save lives, and reduce costs.

Our intention is to revise the book every 2 years. We therefore welcome comments, which will be incorporated into the next edition. Remarks may be sent to:

Dr. Timothy Brewer
International Society for Infectious Diseases
181 Longwood Avenue
Boston, MA 02115 USA
Fax: 617 731 1541
e-mail: ISIDbos@aol.com

We wish to thank all our colleagues and friends for their contributions.

J-P. Butzler, R. Wenzel
Co-Chairs of the ISID Infection Control Working Group

Contents

CHAPTER 1

IMPORTANCE OF INFECTION CONTROL

Shaheen Mehtar, MBBS, FRCP

The quality of a hospital's or health center's infection control program is a reflection of the overall standard of care provided by that institution. Good infection control programs reduce nosocomial infections, length of stay in the hospital, and costs associated with hospitalization.

Historically, infection control practices, in one form or another, have existed since surgeons such as Lister recognized the significance of bacteria in producing postoperative wound infection. In the early 1970s, the first infection control nurse was appointed in the United Kingdom. This marked the beginning of an era: the recognition of infection control as a specialty in its own right. In some countries, medical insurance companies pressured health services to reduce infection rates, and this in turn has lead to an increase in infection control programs.

Countries with developed health care systems have responded to the need to control hospital infections, reflected in escalating costs of hospitalization and increased length of stay in patients with infections, by establishing infection control programs that span the spectrum of hospital practice and clinical activity and provide a means of evaluating the outcome of infection by clinical audit. Good programs develop standards for quality care of patients that are integrated into clinical practice. By making governments and communities aware of the reduced morbidity and mortality from infections, as well as the costs savings resulting from infection control programs, support for these vital functions is enhanced.

In developing health care programs, however, the situation is different. Infection control programs are either in their infancy or nonexistent. Individual hospitals and physicians struggle to establish programs with little support from their respective governments. Infection control is considered a low priority where health programs are subject to severe budgetary constraints, and a commitment to provide adequate clinical care is difficult to fulfill. Problems such as high rates of infection, antibiotic-resistant bacteria which are difficult to treat within the available resources, and a lack of sound surveillance are further multiplied by overcrowding in hospitals, lack of private resources to supplement medical care, and lack of coherent policies. It is with this perspective in mind that infection control programs should be established within the available resources in such countries. An emphasis on rural health care units such as clinics at primary care level can bring infection control programs within the scope of practice of all health care workers.

Why Should There Be Infection Control Programs?

Infection control programs are cost effective. A number of studies have shown that establishing infection control guidelines based on scientific evidence results in considerable savings. The SENIC study demonstrated that good infection control programs result in real savings and improved health care for the patients. Clinical care protocols and appropriate antibiotic use reduce infection, thus decreasing the length of stay in hospitals (the single-most expensive part of medical care).

Infection control programs reduce morbidity and mortality. Infection control teams are particularly helpful for preventing outbreaks caused by multidrug-resistant organisms such as methicillin-resistant *Staphylocccus aureus* (MRSA) or gram-negative bacilli. A significant contribution has been made in high-risk areas, such as intensive care units (ICUs), where infection rates have been reduced by good infection control practice. These patients are usually sicker, require more invasive therapy, medical intervention, and aggressive therapy, and are therefore at higher risk for acquiring infections.

Detecting Infections in a Health Care Unit

In order to reduce nosocomial infections, it is essential to first establish the extent of the problem. This requires identification of the prevalent types of pathogens, antibiotic resistance or sensitivity patterns amongst bacteria, and routes of spread or cross-infection. Continuous or targeted surveillance is used to determine the extent of nosocomial infections that are occurring. Continuous surveillance requires staff, data capture systems, and well-organized reporting systems, ideally in all areas of a health care facility. It is effective in showing trends in antibiotic resistance patterns, the effect of long-term interventions, and for acquiring baseline data upon which infection control programs may be established on a scientific basis. As with any surveillance system, collecting information is only useful if improvements are made based on good information. In some aspects, the results are retrospective and may not reflect immediate changes which occur with outbreaks of infection.

Targeted surveillance is used to pick up information about an area or a possible outbreak. The resources required are more manageable, and in most instances, the outcome is immediately visible. It is an effective way of educating staff and effecting unit infection control policies in a short time. The drawbacks are that overall baseline data may be lacking when continuous surveillance has not been done, and that surveillance is stopped after the episode is over.

When starting an infection control program, a short period of time should be spent on continuous surveillance to establish baseline data, followed by targeted surveillance of high-risk areas.

Utilizing Surveillance Information

It is essential to understand the sources of infection and routes of spread to establish simple and sensible infection control measures. Once these are fully understood, interventions which contain the spread of pathogens can be instituted.

Good infection control practice can usually contain most infections by simple measures. This last point should be emphasized, particularly in developing countries where expensive facilities may not be available.

Infection control programs are only as effective as the understanding of the staff who implement them. A good infection control program is underpinned by a dedicated and knowledgeable infection control team, in which the doctors and nurses involved directly in infection control are responsive to the needs of the staff and patients, and are prepared to learn, teach, and acknowledge the achievements of the program.

CHAPTER 2

HANDWASHING

Richard P. Wenzel, MD, MSc

Key Issue: Handwashing is the most important infection control practice by hospital staff to minimize the transmission of infection between patients.

Known Facts

- Simple soap-and-water handwashing will remove almost all transient gram-negative rods in 10 seconds.
- Regretably, most doctors and nurses in intensive care units do not wash their hands after each patient contact. On average, compliance with recommended handwashing is only 40% in ICUs.

Controversial Issues

- Alcohol may be as good as or better than simple soap-and-water handwashing for removing transient bacteria.
- Chlorhexidine may be better than nonmedicated soaps for removal of transient gram-positive organisms.

Suggested Practice

- Ten-second handwashing is recommended after all patient encounters or when going from a contaminated part of a patient, such as a wound dressing, to a clean site, such as a medical device (e.g., vascular catheter), on the same patient.

Summary: In the mid-1800s, one of the major causes of death of young women delivering babies was "puerperal sepsis." We now know that this infection was caused by group A beta-hemolytic *Streptococcus pyogenes*.

In 1846, Dr. Ignaz Semmelweis, a young obstetrician, noted that coincident with the introduction of the gross autopsy, deaths from puerperal sepsis increased. He recognized the practice of physicians and medical students examining women who died

Table 2.1 Data—Lying in Hospital 1846

	Ward I	Ward II
Caregivers	Physicians and Medical Students	Midwives
Mortality from puerperal sepsis	8%	2%
Mortality after handwashing introduction	1.5%	—

of puerperal sepsis and then going directly to the wards where they performed repeated examinations of women in labor.

Semmelweis noted that on wards where midwives delivered babies, few mothers died of puerperal sepsis. He knew that midwives did not witness autopsies. Semmelweis reasoned that something was carried from the autopsy room to the wards on the hands of physicians and students. He introduced a simple handwashing regimen, and rates of death due to puerperal sepsis fell (Table 2.1).

In the 1970s, Katherine Sprunt showed that a brief handwash with any soap and water removes almost all transient gram-negative rods on the hands of nurses who had just changed a baby's diaper. In the 1980s, Ojajarvi from Finland showed that some gram-positive organisms may not be as easily washed off as gram-negative organisms. Alcohol, or chlorhexidine, if available, may be somewhat better for the removal of gram-positive bacteria. Nevertheless, a careful 10-second handwash with any soap and water is remarkably effective in reducing carriage of bacteria.

Many studies of alcohol suggest that it is the most rapidly active agent for cleaning hands. In some cultures, chlorhexidine or other soaps may be more acceptable to nursing and medical personnel. Regardless of the agent, the main point is to improve compliance of simple handwashing between patient contacts.

Reference

Doebbeling BN, Stanley GL, Sheetz CT, Pfaller MA, Houston AK, Annis L, Wenzel RP. Comparative efficacy of alternative handwashing agents in reducing nosocomial infections in intensive care units. N Engl J Med 1992;327: 88–93.

CHAPTER 3

ISOLATION OF COMMUNICABLE DISEASES

M. Sigfrido Rangel-Frausto, MD, MSc

Key Issue: Isolation procedures are the most effective way of stopping the dissemination of an infection from patient to patient, and from patient to health care workers (HCWs).

Known Facts: Isolation procedures are needed by 7 to 12% of patients admitted to hospitals. However, only 17 to 43% of patients who should be isolated are isolated. Only 50% of isolation procedures are maintained for those started on isolation.

- Transmission of nosocomial pathogens is due to three basic mechanisms:
  1. Contact, which involves skin-to-skin contact and the direct physical transfer of microorganisms from one patient to another or from an HCW. Direct contact examples are handshaking, bathing patients, etc. Indirect contact refers to contact with an inanimate surface contaminated with microorganisms. For example, contaminated stethoscopes, thermometers, etc.
  2. Droplet, whereby pathogens are spread by respiratory droplets produced during coughing, sneezing, talking, or during invasive procedures such as bronchoscopy. Respiratory droplets larger than 5 microns (μm) do not last very long in the air and usually travel short distances. Most of the time, close contact (usually less than 1 m) is necessary for transmission to occur.
  3. Airborne, whereby this type of transmission is produced by droplets less than 5 μm. Droplets may remain suspended in the air for long periods and travel long distances. They are produced by coughing, talking, sneezing, or by procedures such as bronchoscopy or suctioning. Because

of their airborne nature, they can infect susceptible hosts several meters away from they are produced.

- Additional mechanisms for the transmission of infectious agents include the contamination of the water supply, equipment, solutions, needles, multiple-dose vials, or other articles used by more than one patient.

Suggested Practice: All patients receiving care in hospitals or doctor offices, irrespective of their diagnoses, must be treated in such a manner as to minimize the risk of transmission of any kind of microorganisms from patient to HCW, from HCW to patient, and from patient to HCW to patient. These precautions are known as standard precautions, and they are an improvement on universal precautions and body substance isolation.

- Hands should be washed after all patient contact, irrespective of whether gloves were worn. Handwashing should take place immediately after gloves are removed, before and between patient contacts, and any time one handles blood, body fluids, secretions or excretions, or potentially contaminated items or equipment.
- Gloves should be worn if touching blood, body fluids, secretions, excretions, or contaminated objects. Gloves should be worn in case of touching mucous membranes or broken skin. Gloves must always be changed between patients. After wound dressing changes or other contact with dirty sites, gloves must be changed before touching clean sites on the same patient. Handwashing should be performed after removing gloves. Gloves do not substitute for handwashing.
- Mask and eye protection should be worn to protect mucous membranes during procedures that are likely to result in splashing of blood, body fluids, secretions, or excretions.
- A gown should be worn to protect skin and clothing during procedures that are likely to result in splashing of blood, body fluids, secretions, or excretions. Gowns also may be worn during the care of patients infected with pathogens

such as methicillin-resistant *Staphylococcus aureus* (MRSA) or VRE to reduce the probability of their transmission within the hospital or clinic, or to other patients or HCWs. Gowns are removed before leaving the patient's room and hands are washed.

- Special care must be taken to prevent the exposure of patients, HCWs, or visitors to contaminated materials or equipment. Reusable equipment should be cleaned and sterilized before reuse. Directions for correct cleaning, disinfection, or sterilization should be followed to prevent transmission of infectious pathogens with reuse.
- Soiled linen should be transported in a bag. If the bag is sturdy and the article can be placed in the bag without contaminating the outside of the bag, one bag may be used; otherwise, two bags are used.
- Sharp instruments and needles should be handled with care. When possible, never recap. If recapping is necessary, do not use both hands; rather, use the one-handed technique or a mechanical device to recap safely. *Never remove, bend, break, or manipulate needles from syringes by hand.* Used needles, scalpel blades, and other sharp items should be placed in appropriated puncture-resistant containers. Containers should be close and visible.
- No special precautions are needed for dishes, glasses, cups, and eating utensils. Disposable or reusable dishes can be used in patients on isolation precautions. Hot water and detergents in hospitals are sufficient to decontaminate these articles.
- Rooms, cubicles, and bedside equipment should be appropriately cleaned. In addition to cleaning, adequate disinfection of bedside equipment and environmental surfaces is indicated for certain pathogens such as *Clostridium difficile* and *Enterococcus*.

In addition to these standard precautions, patients suspected of having certain pathogens should be isolated accordingly.

Contact Isolation

Room. Provide a private room, if possible. When private rooms are not available, place the patient with another patient infected with the same microorganism but with no other infection (cohorting).

Gloves. Nonsterile gloves should be worn when entering the room. During patient contact, change gloves after contact with infective material. Remove gloves before leaving the room, and wash hands immediately with an antimicrobial agent or a waterless antiseptic agent. Be sure not to touch potentially contaminated surfaces, equipment, or utensils before leaving the room.

Gown. Gowns (clean, nonsterile) should be worn when entering the room. Remove the gown before leaving the patient's environment, and be careful not to contaminate your clothes.

Patient Transport. Limit patient transport to only that deemed absolutely necessary. During transport, always maintain isolation precautions.

Patient-Care Equipment. When possible, limit the use of non-critical patient-care equipment to a single patient.

Droplet Isolation (droplets larger than 5 microns)

Room. Arrange a private room, if possible, or cohorting with a patient with the same active infection. If not, maintain distance of at least 1 m between infected patient and other patients and visitors. The door should remain open.

Mask. Masks are worn if within less than 1 m of the patient. However, it may be easier to remember to put on the mask upon entering the room.

Patient Transport. Limit patient transport; if transport is necessary, maintain isolation at all times.

Airborne Isolation (droplets smaller than 5 microns)

Room. These patients need a private room where the air flows from the hall into the room (negative air pressure), with 6 to 12 changes per hour and appropriate discharge of air outdoors. Negative air pressure can be created by placing a fan in the window and exhausting the air to the outside. High-efficiency filtration is necessary if the air is circulated in other areas of the hospital. Keep the door closed.

Mask. Respiratory protection should be worn when entering the room; an N95 (N category at 95% efficiency) meets the CDC performance for a tuberculosis respirator.

Patient Transport. Limit movement and transport of the patient. Patients need to wear a mask when they are transported out of their room.

Summary: Contact precautions should be used in suspected cases of diarrhea, respiratory infections (particularly bronchiolitis and croup), or when the patient may be infected or colonized by multidrug-resistant organisms (including history of infection or colonization). Skin, wound, or urinary tract infection in a patient with a recent hospital stay or nursing home stay may be due to multidrug-resistant organisms. Others needing contact precautions include patients with abscesses or draining wounds, skin infections including diphtheria, herpes simplex, impetigo, pediculosis, scabies, zoster, viral/hemorrhagic conjunctivitis, and viral infections such as Ebola, Lassar, and Marburg.

Droplet precautions should be used for patients with invasive *Haemophilus influenzae* type B disease, invasive *Neisseria meningitidis* disease, respiratory infections such as diphtheria, Mycoplasma pneumonia, pertussis, pneumonic plague, streptococcal pharyngitis or scarlet fever in young patients, and viral infections caused by adenovirus, influenza, mumps, parvovirus B19, or rubella.

For patients with infections with respiratory droplets smaller than 5 microns, such as tuberculosis, airborne precautions should be used. Other infections which require airborne precautions include measles and varicella (including disseminated zoster). Patients with possible tuberculosis, such as patients with cough, fever, a pulmonary infiltrate in an HIV-negative patient, or any lung location infiltrate in an HIV-positive patient or patient at high risk for HIV infection, should be placed in airborne precautions until tuberculosis can be excluded or treated.

References

Centers for Disease Control and Prevention. Guidelines for preventing transmission of tuberculosis in health-care facilities. Morb Mortal Wkly Rep 1993;143:1–32

Doebbeling BN, Wenzel RP. The direct costs of universal precautions in a teaching hospital. JAMA 1990;264:2083–7.

Edmond MB, Wenzel RP, Pasculle AW. Vancomycin-resistant *Staphylococcus aureus*: perspectives on measures needed for control. Ann Intern Med 1996;124:329–34.

Garner JS. Centers for Disease Control and Prevention. Guideline for isolation precautions for hospitals. Infect Control Hosp Epidemiol 1996;17:53–80.

Hospital Infection Control Practices Advisory Committee. Recommendations for preventing the spread of vancomycin resistance. Infect Control Hosp Epidemiol 1995;16:105–13.

CHAPTER 4

Sterilization and Use of Sterile Products

Günter Kampf, MD, and Constanze Wendt, MD, MS

Key Issue: Critical medical devices must be sterilized and kept from being contaminated before use to avoid infections in patients exposed to them.

Known Facts
- The success of a sterilization procedure must be monitored using biologic indicators.
- An item should not be used if its sterility is questionable, e.g., if its package is punctured, torn, or wet.

Controversial Issues
- The shelf life of sterile items remains unclear.

Suggested Practice
- Steam sterilization should be used for all items that will not be damaged by heat, pressure, or moisture.
- Biologic monitoring of sterilization procedures should be performed regularly, e.g., once a week.
- Shelf life and expiration-dating policies must be based on packaging materials used and facilities for storage.
- Medical devices or patient-care equipment that enter normally sterile tissue or the vascular system, or through which blood flows, are the so-called critical items. Examples of critical items are surgical instruments, urinary or vascular catheters, or needles. Critical items pose a high risk of infection if they are contaminated with microorganisms. Therefore, they must be sterile.
- Cleaning, disinfection, and sterilization of patient-care supplies should be performed in a central processing department to make quality control easier.

- The central processing area should be divided into several areas including a cleaning and decontamination area, a packaging area, and areas for sterilization and storage of sterile supplies that are separated by physical barriers. Ideally, the temperature of all areas should be maintained between 18°C and 22°C, the relative humidity should be maintained between 35% and 70%, and the air flow should be directed from clean areas to relatively soiled areas.
- Because effective sterilization of critical medical equipment depends upon reduction of the bioburden, before beginning the sterilization process all items should be thoroughly cleaned. Manual cleaning of contaminated items can expose personnel to bloodborne pathogens and other potentially harmful microorganisms and should be avoided.
- Alternatives are ultrasonic cleaning, dishwasher, washer-decontaminator machines, or washer-sterilizers.
- Disinfectant/detergent agents are used increasingly for pre-soaking of contaminated items. However, these agents may damage the instruments, and furthermore, personnel may get a false sense of security since disinfection cannot be accomplished if gross soilage is present. Thus, all items should be considered contaminated and need to be handled with gloves.
- All items to be sterilized should be wrapped or packed to avoid recontamination after the sterilization process. Wrapping materials should
  1. provide a seal of proven integrity,
  2. be free of pinholes,
  3. be durable enough to resist tears and punctures,
  4. not delaminate when opened,
  5. allow printing and labelling,
  6. not generate nonviable particles,
  7. be compatible with the sterilization process, and
  8. be inexpensive, impervious to bacteria, sealable before sterilization, and flexible enough to allow swift wrapping and unwrapping.

Commonly used wrapping materials are 140-thread-count muslin, Kraft paper, nonwoven wraps, and paper/plastic peel-down packages. When single-wrapped sterile packages are used, the contents may be contaminated from the exterior surface upon opening. Therefore, items to be sterilized should be wrapped in two thicknesses of paper or nonwoven fabric.

- Various methods of sterilization are available for hospitals: steam sterilization, dry heat sterilization, and gas sterilization using ethylene oxide, formaldehyde, or vapor phase hydrogen peroxide. Ionizing radiation is another method which is used mainly for industrial sterilization of single-use items. The advantages and disadvantages of each method are summarized in Table 4.1.
- Monitoring the sterilization process is an essential quality assessment procedure for infection control. Physical monitoring is the observation of sterilizer functioning (e.g., temperature, pressure, time). Any deviation from the expected readings should alert the operator to potential problems. Chemical monitoring describes color or physical change indicators that monitor exposure to sterilizing agents or conditions. Biological monitoring is the most important check on sterilizer function. The CDC recommends monitoring of steam autoclaves in hospitals at least weekly. *Bacillus stearothermophilus* spores should be used as biologic indicators for heat sterilizers and *Bacillus subtilis* var. *niger* or var. *globigii* spores for ethylene oxide sterilizers. Every load containing implantable objects should be monitored with a spore test. It is recommended that sterilizer loads containing implantables or intravascular devices be quarantined until the spore test has been reported as negative.
- An optimal sterile storage area is adjacent to the sterilization area and protects the sterile products against dust, moisture, insects, vermin, and temperature and humidity extremes. Sterile items should be positioned such that packaging is not crushed, bent, compressed, or punctured. The term "shelf life"

Table 4.1 Advantages and Disadvantages of Various Sterilization Methods

Method	Advantages	Disadvantages
Steam sterilization	Most common sterilization process in health care facilities Safe for environment and health care workers Short sterilization time Nontoxic Inexpensive No aeration necessary	Success of sterilization can be impaired by trapped air, grossly wet materials, and decreased steam quality Heat- and moisture-sensitive components can be damaged
Dry heat sterilization	Low corrosiveness Deep penetration in the material Safe for the environment No aeration necessary	Requires long sterilization time Requirements of different countries regarding temperature and cycle time are conflicting Heat-labile components can be damaged
100% Ethylene oxide (ETO)	Penetrates packaging materials and many plastics Compatible with most medical materials Simple to operate and monitor	Requires aeration time Small sterilization chamber ETO is toxic, a probable carcinogen, and flammable ETO cartridges need storage in flammable liquid storage cabinet
Hydrogen peroxide plasma sterilization	Low process temperature No aeration necessary Safe for environment and health care worker No toxic residuals Simple to operate, install, and monitor	Cellulose, linens, and liquids cannot be processed Small sterilization chamber Medical devices with long or narrow lumen cannot be processed Requires synthetic packaging
Formaldehyde	Formaldehyde is not flammable or explosive Compatible with most medical materials	Potential for residual formaldehyde on the surface Formaldehyde is toxic and allergenic Requires long sterilization time Long processing time due to removal of formaldehyde after sterilization

is defined as the period during which sterility can be maintained. In the literature, storage times between 2 days and an indefinite period have been reported, but in most instances wrapping materials and storage conditions were not considered. In conclusion, loss of sterility is considered event related (e.g., by the frequency and method of handling and storage area conditions) and not time related. Sterile products transported to the operating rooms and other areas within the hospital should be provided with an additional outer dust-protection cover that can be removed before the items are taken into the clean zone.

References

Cardo DM, Drake A. Central sterile supply. In: Mayhall CG, editor. Hospital epidemiology and infection control. Baltimore, MD: Williams and Wilkins; 1996. p. 799–805.

Garner JS, Favero MS. CDC guideline for handwashing and hospital environmental control, 1985; Supercedes guideline for hospital environmental control published in 1981. Infect Control 1986; 4:231–43.

Keene JH. Sterilization and pasteurization. In: Mayhall, CG, editor. Hospital epidemiology and infection control. Baltimore, MD: Williams and Wilkins; 1996. p. 937–46.

CHAPTER 5

DISINFECTION OF MEDICAL EQUIPMENT

Constanze Wendt, MD, MS

Key Issue: Infections due to improperly decontaminated medical equipment occur frequently and are preventable.

Known Facts
- The level of disinfection needed depends on the item and its intended use.
- Sterilization of all medical equipment is unnecessary and expensive.

Controversial Issues
- Identifying the best method for disinfecting heat-sensitive critical equipment, such as laparoscopes.
- Whether disposable items can or should be disinfected.

Suggested Practice
- Equipment or items that go into the body, through tissue, or have blood or IV fluids flow through them must be sterilized; these are critical items. Semicritical items, which come in contact with mucous membranes or nonintact skin, must be high-level disinfected. Noncritical items, which come in contact with intact skin, can be intermediate-level disinfected.
- Before a disinfection procedure for a medical device can be selected, it must be determined whether that device needs sterilization or disinfection. Though the term **disinfection** is often confused with the term **sterilization**, the two procedures have important differences.

  Sterilization is the complete elimination of all microbial life including resistant bacterial spores. Sterilization is an absolute state, not a relative one. Sterilization can be accomplished by the use of steam under pressure, dry heat, ethylene oxide gas, and liquid chemicals. Liquid chemical sterilization has a higher risk of failure than the other procedures because the devices to be sterilized are not wrapped before sterilizing and the toxic germicides used for sterilization must be rinsed off before use.

Disinfection of equipment or surfaces is the elimination of nearly all recognized pathogenic organisms but not necessarily all microbial forms (such as highly resistant bacterial spores). Disinfection can be accomplished by the use of liquid chemicals or wet pasteurization.

- Based on the risk of infection in patients, three categories of medical devices can be distinguished: 1) critical instruments or devices; 2) semicritical instruments or devices; and 3) noncritical instruments or devices.

Critical items are those which enter the bloodstream or normally sterile body areas, e.g., surgical instruments, implants, and cardiac catheters. If critical instruments are contaminated with any microorganism, a substantial risk of infection exists. Therefore, instruments or devices of this category must be sterile. Of special concern are heat-labile critical items that cannot be easily sterilized, such as laparoscopes. Ethylene oxide sterilization or sterilization by liquid chemicals is very time consuming, forcing some hospitals to perform high-level disinfection for this kind of instruments. This procedure does not completely destroy bacterial endospores, increasing the risk of infection.

Semicritical items come in contact with mucous membranes or nonintact skin (e.g., respiratory-therapy equipment, bronchoscopes, endoscopes). Semicritical instruments must be correctly cleaned and should undergo a disinfection process that eradicates all microorganisms and most bacterial spores.

Noncritical items have contact only with intact skin (e.g., blood pressure cuffs, stethoscopes, bedpans). These items need not be sterile or free of bacterial endospores.

- Depending on the type of the medical device and its use, high-level disinfection (HLD), intermediate-level disinfection (ILD), or low-level disinfection (LLD) can be used (Table 5.1).

Table 5.1 Methods of Sterilization and Disinfection

	Sterilization		Disinfection		
	Critical Items (will enter tissue or vascular system or blood will flow through them)		High-Level (semicritical items; will come in contact with mucous membranes or nonintact skin)	Intermediate-Level (some semicritical items and noncritical items)	Low-Level (noncritical items; will come in contact with intact skin)
Object	Procedure	Exposure Time (hr)	Procedure (exposure time ≥20 min)	Procedure (exposure time ≤10 min)	Procedure (exposure time ≤10 min)
Smooth, hard surface	Heat sterilization	MR	Glutaraldehyde (2%)	Sodium hypochlorite	Ethyl or isopropyl alcohol (70–90%)
	Ethylene oxide gas	MR	6% stabilized hydrogen peroxide	Ethyl or isopropyl alcohol (70–90%)	Sodium hypochlorite
	Glutaraldehyde (2%)	MR	Peracetic acid	Phenolic solutions	Iodophor
	6% stabilized hydrogen peroxide	6	Wet pasteurization at 75°C for 30 min, after detergent cleaning	Iodophor	Phenolic solution
	Peracetic acid	MR	Sodium hypochlorite		Quaternary ammonium solution
Rubber tubing and catheters and polyethylene tubing and catheters	Heat sterilization	MR	Glutaraldehyde (2%)		
	Ethylene oxide gas	MR	6% stabilized hydrogen peroxide		
	Glutaraldehyde (2%)	MR	Peracetic acid		
	6% stabilized hydrogen peroxide	6	Wet pasteurization at 75°C for 30 min. after detergent cleaning		
	Peracetic acid	MR			

Table 5.1 continued

Lensed instruments	Ethylene oxide gas	MR	Glutaraldehyde (2%)
	Glutaraldehyde (2%)	MR	6% stabilized hydrogen peroxide
	6% stabilized hydrogen peroxide	6	Peracetic acid
	Peracetic acid	MR	
Thermometers (oral and rectal)			Iodophor (do not mix rectal and oral thermometers at any stage of processing)
Hinged instruments	Heat sterilization	MR	Glutaraldehyde (2%)
	Ethylene oxide gas	MR	6% stabilized hydrogen peroxide
	Glutaraldehyde (2%)	MR	Peracetic acid
	6% stabilized hydrogen peroxide	6	
	Peracetic acid	MR	

Adapted from Simmons BP: Guidelines for hospital infection control. Am J Infect Control 1983;11:97–115 and Rutala WA. APIC guidelines for selection and use of disinfectants. Am J Infect Control 1996;24:313–42.
MR = Manufacturer's recommendations

HLD destroys all microorganisms with the exception of high numbers of bacterial spores. It should be used for all semicritical items. Glutaraldehyde, chlorine dioxide, 6% hydrogen peroxide, or peracetic acid-based formulations can be used to achieve HLD. These chemicals also can be used as sterilizing agents if the time in the disinfectant is long enough.

ILD destroys vegetative bacteria including *Mycobacterium tuberculosis*, most viruses, and most fungi but not necessarily bacterial spores. Small nonlipid viruses (e.g., enterovirus, rhinovirus) may be more resistant to germicides, but large lipid viruses, such as adenoviruses, hepatitis B virus, or human immunodeficiency virus, are usually destroyed by ILD. ILD should be used for noncritical items. It also can be used for some semicritical items such as hydrotherapy tanks used for patients with nonintact skin. Alcohol (70 to 90% ethanol or isopropyl), chlorine compounds, and certain phenolic and iodophor preparations are intermediate-level disinfectants.

LLD destroys most vegetative bacteria, most viruses, and most fungi but not bacterial endospores, mycobacteria, and small nonlipid viruses. It should be used for noncritical items only. Quaternary ammonium compounds and certain iodophor and phenolic formulations are examples of low-level disinfectants.

- The disinfection procedure is affected by a number of factors, including:
  1. The nature of the item to be sterilized. Devices with joints, crevices, or pores in the surface may be hard to clean. Germicides may not penetrate completely to produce sterilization.
  2. Level and type of microbial contamination. Devices contaminated with higher numbers of microorganisms or more resistant microorganisms need longer exposure to germicides than devices that are contaminated with low numbers of microorganisms or with sensitive microorganisms.
  3. Presence of organic debris. Germicides may react with

blood, serum, pus, or other organic material present on the item to be disinfected and lose activity.

4. Concentration of germicide and duration of exposure. Generally, the greater the concentration of germicide, the shorter is the duration of exposure needed for disinfection. Exceptions are iodophors and alcohol, which may lose activity in concentrations higher than those suggested by the manufacturer.

5. Other physical and chemical factors. Temperature, pH, water hardness, and presence of other chemicals such as soap can influence the efficacy of disinfectants. It is crucial that the germicide come in contact with all surfaces of the equipment being disinfected. Air bubbles or inclusions of air in the devices must be strictly avoided.

- Under some circumstances, hospitals may wish to reprocess disposable medical equipment. These circumstances may include interruption of the supply, use of a noncritical device for a purpose that requires sterility, or economy. However, reuse of disposables raises a number of unresolved questions about toxic residues, pyrogens, functional reliability, structural integrity, law, ethics, and risk acceptance. Reprocessing should be avoided unless permission is obtained from the manufacturer along with specific instruction about reprocessing, inspection, and limits of use (see first reference, below).

References

Greene VW. Reuse of disposable devices. In: Mayhall CG, editor. Hospital epidemiology and infection control. Baltimore, MD: Williams and Wilkins; 1996. p. 946–54.

Rutala WA. APIC guideline for selection and use of disinfectants. Am J Infect Control 1996;24:313–42.

CHAPTER 6

IS THE HEALTH CARE WORKER A SOURCE OF TRANSMISSION?

Bradley N. Doebbeling, MD, MS,
and Margreet C. Vos, MD, PhD

Key Issue: Within the hospital, health care workers (HCWs) are often exposed to infections. Any transmissible disease can occur in the hospital setting and may affect HCWs. HCWs are not only at risk of acquiring infections but also of being a source of infection to patients. Therefore, both the patient and the HCW need to be protected from contracting or transmitting nosocomial infections by using recommended infection control measures.

Known Facts

- The infection control objectives of a hospital should be planned by the infection control committee and health services personnel. The focus of the committee and services must be personal hygiene, monitoring of infectious disease outbreaks and exposures and, after identifying infection risks, institution of preventive measures.
- Prevention of infectious diseases in HCWs serves three purposes: the health of the health care worker, the prevention of work restrictions, and the reduction of nosocomial infections.
- Education is an important factor for improving compliance with guidelines and prevention measures. All HCWs need to know about the risk of infection and the route of transmission of pathogens. Personal hygiene is the foundation for preventing transmission of infectious diseases to patients.
- Immunization should be used to protect HCWs from infectious agents such as hepatitis B virus. Preventing infections in HCWs will also prevent transmission of infections from HCWs to patients. Prompt evaluation of and institution of

appropriate control measures for patients with signs and symptoms of transmissible infectious diseases will reduce the risk of hospital-acquired diseases.

• In deciding the type of infection control procedures needed, one must consider the HCW's job, risk of exposure, and the suspected infectious pathogen.

In general, the risk of transmission of an infection depends on the characteristics of microorganisms and on host factors. To assess the risk of transmission, one has to take into account

• the possibility, quality, quantity, and duration of contact with the infectious source;

• the contagiousness of the causative microorganism, including the capability of the microorganism to survive on objects; and

• the procedures and steps taken by HCWs to avoid infection.

Routes of transmission differ for various microorganisms, and the same microorganism may be transmitted by more than one route. A short overview of some of the most important infectious diseases transmitted by HCWs is presented below.

Skin Infections

Staphylococcus Aureus. About one-third of the population are persistent nasal carriers of *S. aureus* (SA), one-third are intermittent carriers, and one-third are not carriers. Other sites of colonization are the perineum, skin, axilla, or hair. People with dermal lesions, such as eczema, are more likely to be carriers. Carriers can spread SA to patients, especially those with wounds, or intravascular or other indwelling catheters. Dissemination of SA is by direct or indirect contact or, less commonly, by skin scales. Health care workers with lesions caused by SA such as boils (even on an occult body area) or other skin lesions are more likely to transmit infection to others than nasal carriers. Depending on the type of work done by the HCW, work restriction can be considered.

During periods of high incidence of staphylococcal disease or epidemics of methicillin-resistant *Staphylococcus aureus* (MRSA), identifying carriers by culturing patients and HCWs can be useful. Carriers can be treated with 2% mupirocin ointment. Mupirocin should not be used for longer than 5 days as resistance can develop. Since muprocin is an important tool to control epidemic spread by eradication of *S. aureus* from nasal carriers, it should not be used to treat wound infections.

Group A *Streptococcus*. Group A *Streptococcus* (GAS) is a well-known pathogen of the skin and pharynx. Other reservoirs include the rectum and the female genital tract. Major modes of transmission are direct contact and large droplets. An increased incidence of wound infections by GAS should be investigated, focusing on carriage by HCWs. Health care workers with overt infection due to GAS should be restricted from work until 24 hours after adequate therapy has been given or until cultures are proven to be negative. Overall, the risk of transmission of GAS from HCW to patients is considered low.

Herpes Simplex. Herpes simplex type I can be transmitted from HCWs to patients through primary or recurrent lesions. Most infections are orofacial and transmitted by direct contact. Saliva also can be infectious. Because the main route of transmission is by contaminated hands after direct contact with the lesion, handwashing and disinfection before and after patient contact are the most important methods for preventing transmission to patients. Herpes simplex lesions of the fingers (herpetic whitlow) are an occupational disease of HCWs due to direct exposure to contaminated fluid such as vaginal secretions or skin lesions. Health care workers with herpetic whitlow must use gloves to prevent the spread of the herpes virus to patients. When caring for patients at risk of severe infection, such as neonates, patients with severe malnutrition, severely burned, or immunocompromised patients, restriction of work of HCWs with herpes infections can be considered.

Enteric Diseases

Acute Diarrhea. Transmission of most microorganisms causing diarrhea in HCWs is by direct or indirect contact. Careful handwashing hygiene, especially after visiting the bathroom, is the most important measure for preventing transmission of these pathogens. Until they are better, health care workers with acute infectious diarrhea should not care for patients. Even after resolution of the acute disease, HCWs may still carry enteric pathogens.

HCWs can be asymptomatic carriers of *Salmonella* spp or *Campylobacter* spp during the convalescent period or a protracted period thereafter. Testing for carriage may be unreliable and is therefore usually limited to food handlers, who are more likely to transmit disease to others. Careful handwashing after using the bathroom and before patient contact will prevent the transmission of enteric pathogens from most carriers. Antibiotic treatment is rarely indicated.

Hepatitis A. Hepatitis A occurs rather infrequently as a nosocomial infection. Prevention of transmission is through maintaining personal hygiene, especially through handwashing.

Respiratory Diseases

Common Cold. The common cold in adults is caused by the parainfluenza virus, adenovirus, rhinovirus, or respiratory syncytial virus. Health care workers are important sources of these viruses to patients.

In general, to prevent nosocomial transmission from HCWs to patients, infected HCWs should wash their hands carefully before patient contact. The use of masks is optional but may be helpful in preventing transmission due to large droplets upon close contact. Routine use of gloves has no additional benefit; even if gloves are used, hands should be washed after gloves are removed.

In most people, viral upper respiratory infections are self-limiting. However, in immunocompromised patients, such as recipients of bone marrow transplants, these infections may progress to severe lower respiratory tract diseases with very high mortality rates. Infection control strategies include identifying, cohorting, and isolating of infected patients and limiting contact of symptomatic HCWs and visitors with at-risk patients. Work restrictions for symptomatic HCWs may be considered.

Education of HCWs about the transmission and control of upper respiratory tract infections as well as the seriousness of these infections to bone marrow transplant patients is an important measure.

Influenza. Influenza epidemics are well known in hospitals. Transmission occurs from HCWs to other HCWs and patients, and from patients to HCWs and other patients. Hospital infection committees should implement an influenza vaccination program each year, several weeks before the influenza season.

Tuberculosis. All HCWs reporting symptoms suggestive of tuberculosis should have a medical examination and a chest radiograph. Suggestive symptoms are cough for more than 3 weeks, persistent fever, and weight loss.

After identifying an HCW suffering from open tuberculosis, a prompt evaluation of all contacts must be instituted. Stringent measures regarding work restrictions are necessary. Health care workers should be receiving effective treatment and have negative sputum smears before returning to work.

Bacille Calmette-Guérin (BCG) vaccination should be considered for all tuberculin skin test negative HCWs, unless previously vaccinated, in countries where tuberculosis is endemic or in hospitals where exposure to infectious TB cases is likely.

Bloodborne Diseases

The management of HCWs infected with bloodborne pathogens has been reviewed by the AIDS/TB committee of the Society for Healthcare Epidemiology of America (SHEA). In general, prevention of infection is based on appropriate infection control procedures to avoid blood contact from patient to HCW and from HCW to patient. The major emphasis is on applying blood precautions, practicing handwashing, minimizing contact with blood or blood-contaminated excretions, and handling all blood as potentially infectious. Education concerning bloodborne pathogens for all health care workers is recommended, not just those who are already infected.

Hepatitis B. Immunization with the hepatitis B virus (HBV) vaccine is the most important measure to prevent infection of the HCW by HBV. Each hospital must develop an immunization strategy. Health care workers with active HBV or those who are carriers of HBV are at risk for transmitting HBV to others. The risk of transmission of HBV is higher than that of the hepatitis C virus or human immunodeficiency virus, as is reflected in 38 outbreaks of HBV by HCW-to-patient transmission in the past 22 years.

Vaginal hysterectomy, major pelvic surgery, and cardiac surgery are associated with HBV transmission despite the use of good infection control procedures. With these surgeries, the chances of needle-stick injuries are presumably greater. Before increased use of infection control interventions, the risk of HBV transmission was also associated with dental procedures. The presence of hepatitis B e antigen (HBeAg) in the HCW concerned in transmission was almost always the case except in one instance. Another route of transmission can be by hepatitis B surface antigen (HBsAg)-positive HCWs with exudative dermatitis on body areas that may come in contact with patients.

In the SHEA position paper, it is recommended that HBeAg-positive HCWs should be restricted from practice of gynecologic or cardiac surgery or performing dental procedures. The risk of transmission to patients, despite appropriate use of infection control measures, was considered to be too high. Furthermore, HBV-positive HCWs should double-glove routinely for all procedures in which their blood or body fluids may come in contact with patients.

When patients are exposed to an HCW's blood or body fluids, testing of the HCW for bloodborne pathogens should be done.

Human Immunodeficiency Virus (HIV) and Hepatitis C Virus (HCV)

The risk of transmission of HIV is probably 100 times lower than hepatitis B, with that of HCV being somewhere between HIV and HBV.

Health care workers known to be infected with HIV or HCV are strongly recommended to follow universal precautions as recommended in their hospital to minimize the risk of infection to others. Using double gloves for procedures is recommended. HIV- and HCV-infected HCWs should not be prohibited from patient care activities solely on the basis of their infection. Health care workers need not be screened routinely for HIV or HCV infection, except in cases of significant exposure of a patient to the blood or body fluid of an HCW.

AIDS

Health care workers infected with HIV can be infected with HIV-associated pathogens. In turn, these pathogens can be transmissible to patients. Examples are *Mycobacterium tuberculosis*, varicella zoster, and measles by aerogenic spread and *Salmonella* spp, *Cryptosporidium* spp, and all other enteric pathogens via fecal-oral exposure. For prevention of transmission, see the relevant part of this chapter.

Vaccine-Preventable Diseases

Health care workers may be exposed to vaccine-preventable diseases and then, after contracting the disease, be infectious to patients. The Centers for Disease Control and Prevention (CDC) recommends that HCWs be vaccinated or have demonstrated immunity to certain vaccine-preventable diseases. The infection control committee of each hospital has to develop policies requiring proof of immunity or, if needed, offer vaccination. Herd immunity of the hospital community cannot be relied on, and unvaccinated HCWs are a potential risk to patients.

Varicella Zoster. Varicella zoster virus causes varicella or chickenpox in childhood. After years, due to reactivation, the virus can manifest as skin lesions (zoster or shingles), which may be widely disseminated in immunocompromised patients. Those lesions can be infectious to others through direct contact and cause varicella in susceptible persons.

Varicella is one of the most common hospital-acquired diseases among HCWs. It is a highly contagious disease, and exposure to the virus is common in the health care setting. Most persons with a clear history of chickenpox in childhood are probably immune. Persons with a negative history can be immune but should be tested. Susceptible HCWs can acquire infection after exposure to infectious patients. Nonimmune HCWs exposed to varicella should be excluded from work for up to 21 days to ensure that secondary infection has not occurred. If the HCW develops disease, he/she should be excluded from work until all lesions are dry and crusty. Since such a policy regarding work restriction is very expensive, vaccination of all susceptible workers should be done.

Measles. Measles is transmitted by the airborne route. The same strategy as has been recommended for varicella-susceptible HCWs can be followed for susceptible HCWs exposed to measles. Prompt identification of HCWs with rash and fever will help prevent further spread of this virus.

References

AIDS/TB committee of the Society for Healthcare Epidemiology of America. Management of health care worker infected with hepatitis B virus, hepatitis C virus, human immunodeficiency virus or other bloodborne pathogens. Infect Control Hosp Epidemiol 1997;18:347–63.

Bell D, Shapiro CN, Chamberland ME, Ciesielski CA. Preventing bloodborne pathogen transmission from health care workers to patients: the CDC perspective. Surg Clin North Am 1995;75: 1189–1203.

Centers for Disease Control. Update: universal precautions for prevention of transmission of human immunodeficiency virus, hepatitis B virus, and other bloodborne pathogens in health care settings. Morb Mortal Wkly Rep 1988;37;377–82,387–88.

Eltringham I. Mupirocin resistance and methicillin-resistant *Staphylococcus aureus* (MRSA). J Hosp Infect 1997;35:1–8.7.

Garcia R, Raad I, Abi-Said D, Bodey G, Champlin R, Tarrand J, et al. Nosocomial respiratory syncytial virus infections: prevention and control in bone marrow transplant patients. Infect Control Hosp Epidemiol 1997;18:412–6.

Garner J, The Hospital Infection Control Practices Advisory Committee. Guideline for isolation precaution in hospitals. Infect Control Hosp Epidemiol 1996;17:53–80.

Nettleman MD, Schmid M. Controlling varicella in the health care setting: the cost-effectiveness of using varicella vaccine in health care workers. Infect Control Hosp Epidemiol 1997;18:504–8.

Reagan DR, Bradley N, Doebbeling N, Pfaller MA, Sheetz CT, Houston AK, et al. Elimination of coincident *Staphylococcus aureus* nasal and hand carriage with intranasal application of mupirocin calcium ointment. Ann Intern Med 1991;114:101–6.

Wenzel RP, ed. Prevention and control of nosocomial infections. 3rd ed. Baltimore (MD): Williams and Wilkins; 1997.

Wenzel RP, Nettleman MD, Jones RN, Pfaller MA. Methicillin-resistant *Staphylococcus aureus*: implications for the 1990s and effective measures. Am J Med 1991;91:221s–7s.

Williams W, Hospital Infections Program, National Centers for Infectious Diseases, Centers for Disease Control and Prevention. Guideline for infection control in hospital personnel. Atlanta:1983.

CHAPTER 7

PROBLEMS WITH ANTIBIOTIC RESISTANCE

Richard P. Wenzel, MD, MSc

Key Issue: Begun in the 1940s, the antibiotic era is only 50 years old, yet now is challenged by the worldwide incidence of resistance by microorganisms.

Known Facts
- In the community, penicillin-resistant pneumococci and multidrug-resistant tuberculosis are major public health problems. These diseases also have become significant nosocomial pathogens.
- In hospitals throughout the world, there are special problems with methicillin-resistant *Staphylococcus aureus* and coagulase-negative *Staphylococcus*.
- The explosion of infections with vancomycin-resistant *Enterococcus* in hospitals in the United States has been remarkable.
- Resistance of gram-negative rods to quinolones and third-generation cephalosporins continues to increase.

Unless we pay attention to the problem of antibiotic resistance, we will quickly run out of effective therapy. This point is highlighted in the 1997 reports from Japan and the United States of isolated cases of *Staphylococcus aureus* infections due to organisms partially resistant to vancomycin (MIC = 8 µg/ml).

Controversial Issues
- The **causes** of antibiotic resistance are not clearly known, but surely unnecessary use of antibiotics is important. Such high use leads to the selection of resistant organisms. Once a patient has a resistant organism, then the possibility exists for transmission to other patients.
- A second issue is excellent **infection control**—isolation and

handwashing—to minimize spread of antibiotic resistant isolates.

- The third issue is quickly **identifying patients** entering the hospital who might harbor an antibiotic-resistant organism. This requires labeling the charts of patients previously known to be carriers of or infected with an antibiotic-resistant pathogen. When the patient enters the hospital, he or she is automatically placed in appropriate isolation.

Suggested Practice: Three areas for control of this problem are as follows:

1. Minimize the use of antibiotics to limit the selection and emergence of a resistant clone.
2. Maximize good handwashing and isolation practices to limit transmission of any antibiotic-resistant organisms that may emerge in the hospital or enter with a new patient.
3. Develop systems to identify quickly and isolate immediately all new patients who might be carrying an antibiotic-resistant pathogen. This may be accomplished by marking the charts of patients previously known to be carriers or by isolating all patients coming from another facility known to have a high number of antibiotic-resistant organisms.

References

Edmond MB, Wenzel RP, Pasculle AW. Vancomycin-resistant *Staphylococcus aureus*: perspectives on measures needed for control. Ann Intern Med 1996;124:329–34.

Wenzel RP. Preoperative antibiotic prophylaxis. N Engl J Med 1992; 236:337–9.

Wenzel R, Nettleman M, Jones R, Pfaller M. Methicillin-resistant *Staphylococcus aureus*: implications for the 1990s and effective control measures. Am J Med 1991;91:221S–7S.

CHAPTER 8

ORGANIZING AND RECORDING PROBLEMS INCLUDING EPIDEMICS

R. Samuel Ponce de Leon, MD, MSc

Key Issue: Surveillance is the foundation for organizing and maintaining an infection control program.

Known Facts
- Recording reviews, interviewing of nurses and physicians, and reviewing microbiology results give the infection control team an accurate view of the frequency and type of nosocomial infections. At the same time, performing these activities gives the infection control team or nurse a highly visible profile to all services and personnel, which results in changes in clinical practices.
- Frequently visiting the different units allows for the early detection of outbreaks (there being no other way to detect an epidemic in the earliest stage) and provides information necessary to maintaining the functioning of the overall program.
- Ongoing surveillance provides the results needed to conduct a continuous evaluation of the interventions begun by the infection control committee. Based on these results, infection control regulations and policies may need to be changed. Surveillance is the most effective way of maintaining continuous improvement.
- Reporting surveillance results is an essential element for an effective infection control program. Reports to clinical services must be regular, periodic, and presented in a nonantagonistic way to encourage change. For infection control activities to succeed, the program must include personnel dedicated exclusively to surveillance.
- The frequency of nosocomial epidemics in developing countries is higher than that reported in the United States. This

problem can be particularly severe in neonatal intensive care units because

1. the functioning of these units includes multiple invasive devices without organized procedures and policies to prevent infectious complications; and
2. reutilization, without appropriate sterilization, of disposable devices such as catheters, hemodialysis filters, and needles is unavoidable because of financial considerations.

- The organization of a nosocomial infection program should start with the surveillance system. Surveillance is the central activity from which all other related actions are sustained. Surveillance must be active and continuous, in some cases focused on the highest risk areas. The extent of this activity depends on hospital needs and resources.
- Passive surveillance is not an effective method of infection control.
- Surveillance provides information on the type of pathogen, the frequency of nosocomial infections, the location of nosocomial infections, and the trends over time. Periodic reports should be brief and clear. If possible, reports should be evaluated monthly at the infection control committee meeting. The results can be given as ratios and incidence (or incidence density, number of cases/1000 patient-days) for all nosocomial infections, and by site of infection related to the total number of admissions in the period (per month), by service (e.g., intensive care unit, internal medicine, pediatrics, surgery, obstetrics).
- Outbreak surveillance in the hospital relies on day-to-day visits to the clinical areas, the results of the clinical microbiology laboratory, and spontaneous calls from different wards. The system ideally should detect two or three associated cases as soon as they appear, and not after several cases or deaths have occurred.
- Epidemics occur most frequently in intensive care areas. In

developing countries, neonatal intensive care units have the highest risk for nosocomial infections and deaths. These epidemics are most commonly caused by bloodstream infections due to contamination of intravascular lines. Inappropriate handling and storage of multiple vials for small doses of medications to the neonates, the use of glucose infusions, and the lack of handwashing in an overcrowded unit with shortage of personnel and inadequate design are other predisposing factors.

Controversial Issues

- Definitions of nosocomial infections may be controversial. Definitions must be understood as tools for surveillance and will not always agree with the clinician's view. For example, a patient with fever for a few hours and positive blood and catheter tip cultures for *S. epidermidis* should be recorded as a nosocomial infection even if the clinician does not give treatment and the fever disappears with the withdrawal of the line.

- Definitions must be simple and meet hospital purposes. Hospitals without microbiology support can develop definitions based exclusively on clinical data. The Pan-American Health Organization (PAHO) has published a booklet with clinical definitions. The definitions proposed by Wenzel may be useful for hospitals with limited resources.

Summary: In general, hospitalwide surveillance is needed to start a program to identify the highest-risk areas. There is a trend to focus surveillance in high-risk areas, specifically intensive care units, as the efficacy of detecting the more severe nosocomial infections and the most frequent epidemics is very high, as compared to hospitalwide surveillance. However, for hospitals beginning surveillance, it may be better to institute a hospitalwide system in order to know the particular characteristics of their institution. This will also facilitate the collection of endemic rates in every ward. With time, surveillance activities may be limited to high-risk areas.

Control of epidemics requires a reinforcement of general measures of infection control. The infection control team should talk to the personnel on the wards, emphasizing handwashing, isolation practices, and stringent adherence to procedural recommendations. Depending on the characteristics of the outbreak, specific recommendations must be given. A frequent practice when confronting an epidemic is to close the unit and fumigate the area instead of following infection control recommendations. This approach is costly and is not helpful.

General recommendations for surveillance are that

- it must be based on practical definitions
- it must be continuous on wards and the microbiology laboratory
- for every instance of suspected nosocomial infection, forms should be filled out recording diagnosis, age, ward, times of admission and discharge, outcome, type of infection, and etiologic agent
- monthly results of surveillance should be reported to the clinical services in a simple format, and the results presented at the infection control meeting. Decisions to improve control need to be discussed and implemented.

General recommendations in epidemics

- An epidemic is an infection control emergency; measures should be taken as soon as an epidemic is suspected.
- The first step in controlling an epidemic is to reinforce general recommendations of infection control in the ward where the cases are occurring. A case definition is made (e.g., *Enterobacter cloacae* bacteremia in neonates in the neonatal intensive care unit) and then current case rates are compared to previous rates (pre-epidemic period).
- After reviewing cases, additional recommendations should be given to the staff in order to prevent new cases.
- A case-control study should be performed to identify specific risk factors. Maintain frequent communication with the clin-

ical staff in the unit or ward involved and give them all relevant information from your analysis.
- After the analysis you may be able to identify one or several risk factors and make changes to prevent future outbreaks. If not, in most cases the study and interventions should be able to contain the epidemic.

The organization of an infection control program in a hospital with very limited resources requires determination and good relations with the clinical staff. Because a constant goal for most hospitals is cutting costs, explaining the cost benefits of infection control procedures will help get support for the program. It is practical to create a local scenario and to calculate savings and the implicit improvements in the quality of care.

Maintain good channels of communication. Authorities must feel and know that the program is solving problems instead of creating them. The fearful perceptions regarding nosocomial infections must be changed. The attitude of the infection control group should be optimistic and creative; there is always the possibility of improvement, even if the level you reach is not the same as those reported by others.

References

Macias-Hernandez A, Hernandez-Ramos I, Mufioz-Barret J, Vargas Salado E, Guerrero Martinez F, Medina-Valdovinos H, et al. Pediatric primary gram-negative bacteremia: a possible relationship with infusate contamination. Infect Control Hosp Epidemiol 1996;17: 276–80.

Ponce de Leon RS. Nosocomial infections in Latin America: we have to start now. Infect Control 1984;5:511–2.

Ponce de Leon S, Rangel-Frausto S. Organizing for infection control with limited resources. In: Wenzel RP, editor. Prevention and control of nosocomial infections. 3rd ed. Baltimore: William and Wilkins; 1997. p. 85–93.

Wenzel RP. Management principles and the infection control committee. In: Wenzel RP, editor. Prevention and control of nosocomial infections. 2nd ed. Baltimore (MD): Williams and Wilkins; 1993. p. 207–13.

Wenzel RP, Thompson RL, Landry SM, Rusell BS, Miller PJ, Ponce de Leon RS. Hospital-acquired infections in intensive care patients: an overview with emphasis on epidemics. Infect Control 1983;4:371–5.

Zaidi M, Sifuentes J, Bobadilla M, Moncada D, Ponce de Leon RS. Epidemic of *Serratia marcescens* bacteremia and meningitis in a neonatal unit in Mexico City. Infect Control Hosp Epidemiol 1989; 10:14–20.

CHAPTER 9

PATIENT AREAS

Constanze Wendt, MD, MS

Key Issue: The patient environment harbors a number of potential reservoirs for pathogens.

Known Facts: Patients need a clean environment for their uncomplicated recovery.

Controversial Issues
- The extent to which environmental reservoirs contribute to nosocomial infections remains unclear.
- The extent to which germicidal solutions should be used on environmental surfaces as opposed to nongermicidal cleaning methods is also unclear.

Suggested Practice
- Patient areas should be cleaned periodically and after contamination.
- Patient areas should be protected from heavy dust.
- Pathogens stay in the environment most of the time during the hospital treatment of patients. Since the writings of Florence Nightingale in the 19th century, no one has questioned the need for a clean environment for the uncomplicated recovery of hospitalized patients. However, there is legitimate doubt as to the extent to which environmental reservoirs contribute to nosocomial infections.
- It has been demonstrated that some parts of the environment have served as reservoirs for outbreaks of nosocomial infections, e.g., air filters, insulation materials, or surfaces. Other objects and surfaces known to harbor bacteria, such as flowers, toilets, and medical waste have not been clearly linked to nosocomial infections.

Environmental Surfaces

Environmental surfaces have been associated with outbreaks of vancomycin-resistant *Enterococcus* and methicillin-resistant *Staphylococcus aureus* (MRSA). However, these special problems do not justify routine disinfection of hospital floors and furnishings. It has been demonstrated that the rate of nosocomial infections are not significantly different between units cleaned with disinfectants and those units cleaned with detergents. It seems that environmental surfaces are contaminated by patients, not the other way around.

Routine cleaning of environmental surfaces with detergents is sufficient in most circumstances. In case of outbreaks, especially outbreaks due to resistant microorganisms found in the environment, additional cleaning with a disinfection solution may be indicated. Disinfecting surfaces is not a substitute for infection control measures to contain the outbreak.

Hospital Toilet

Culturing of hospital toilets has demonstrated that frequency and level of contamination is usually low, making the toilets an uncommon source of hospital infections. However, in units for mentally impaired adults, young children, or neurologically impaired patients, heavy soiling with feces may occur resulting in cross-infections between patients.

Surfaces of hospital toilets should be cleaned with a disinfecting solution. The bowl should be cleaned with a scouring powder and a brush but disinfectants should not be poured into the bowl.

Flowers and Plants

Water of cut flowers may yield high numbers of microorganisms including *Acinetobacter* spp, *Klebsiella* spp, *Enterobacter* spp, *Pseudomonas* spp, *Serratia marcescens*, and *Flavobacterium*.

Although it has never been demonstrated that microorganisms from cut flowers or potted plants were linked with nosocomial infections, cut flowers and potted plants should be avoided in rooms of immunocompromised and intensive care unit patients. In other units, flowers should be handled by support staff with no patient contact, or gloves should be worn for flower handling. Antibacterial agents, e.g., 0.01% to 0.02% chlorhexidine or 10 ml of 1% hypochlorite can be added to the vase water.

Soiled Linen

Every patient should have clean, freshly laundered bed linen. Because it has been demonstrated that the handling of used bed linen may increase the concentration of airborne microorganisms, it has been suggested to disinfect blankets. However, there are no data to support the additional cost and workload needed to disinfect blankets.

Soiled linen should be handled as little as possible and with minimum agitation. They should not be sorted or prerinsed in patient care areas. Linens soiled with blood or body fluids should be deposited and transported in bags that prevent leakage.

Construction Projects

The relation between construction projects and fungal infections has been demonstrated frequently. Thus, careful control measures are needed during hospital construction projects to prevent these infections.

These measures should include erection of physical barriers and temporary shutdown of ventilation systems. If possible, air flow of ventilation systems should be rerouted to protect sensitive areas. Traffic flow patterns for construction personnel should be defined and separated from those of patients and health care workers.

Table 9.1 Possible Reservoirs of Infectious Agents in the Environment and Modes of Control

Reservoir	Associated Pathogen	Control
Patient rooms		
Air filters	*Aspergillus*	Replace soiled filters periodically
False ceilings	*Rhizopus*	Barrier protection during reconstruction
Fireproof material	*Aspergillus*	Add fungicide to moist material
Air fluidized beds	–	Follow manufacturer's recommendation
Mattresses	*Pseudomonas, Acinetobacter*	Use intact plastic cover; disinfect between patients
Carpets	–	Prudent to avoid in areas of heavy soiling
Bathroom		
Faucet aerators	*Pseudomonas*	No precautions necessary
Sinks	*Pseudomonas*	Use separate sinks for handwashing and disposal of contaminated fluids
Tub immersion	*Pseudomonas*	Add germicide to water, drain, and disinfect after each use
Urine-measuring device	*Serratia*	Disinfect between patients, good handwashing
Routinely used medical equipment		
ECG electrodes	*S. aureus,* Gram-negative rods	Disinfect after use or use disposable leads
Stethoscopes	*Staphylococcus*	Prudent to clean periodically with alcohol
Electronic thermometers	*C. difficile*	Probe cover; disinfect each day and when visibly contaminated
Thermometers (glass)	*Salmonella*	Disinfect between use
Plaster	*Pseudomonas, Bacillus, Clostridium, Cunninghamella*	Use judiciously in immunocompromised patients or over nonintact skin
Elasticized bandages	*Zygomycetes*	Avoid in immunocompromised patients or over nonintact skin

Table 9.1 continued

Reservoir	Associated Pathogen	Control
Other possible sources		
Chutes	*Pseudomonas, Staphylococcus*	Proper design and placement
Contaminated germicides	*Pseudomonas*	Avoid extrinsic contamination and seek manufacturer's microbicidal efficiency verification of claims
Ice baths	*Staphylococcus, Ewingella*	Avoid direct contact with ice to cool IV solutions/syringes; use closed system for thermodilution
Water baths	*Pseudomonas, Acinetobacter*	Add germicide to water bath or use plastic overwrap
Pigeon droppings	*Aspergillus*	Filter all hospital air; maintain filter efficiency
Pets	*Salmonella*	Prudent to avoid in hospital setting (except seeing-eye dogs)

Adapted from Weber DJ, Rutala WA. Environmental issues and nosocomial infection. In: Wenzel RP, editor. Prevention and control of nosocomial infections. 3rd ed. Baltimore (MD): Williams and Wilkins; 1997. p. 491–514.

Infective Solid Waste

Infective solid waste may come from patients under isolation precautions, laboratories, and from pathology. Sharp items, blood, and blood products should also be considered infective.

There is no evidence linking infective waste with nosocomial infections in patients. Nevertheless, personnel handling infectious waste should be informed of the potential health and safety hazards. If necessary, the waste should be transported in sealed impervious containers and stored in areas accessible only to personnel involved in the disposal process.

▌ Other Reservoirs

Other possible reservoirs of nosocomial pathogens are summarized in Table 9.1.

References

Maki DG, Alvarado CJ, Hassemer CA and Zilz MA. Relation of the inanimate hospital environment to endemic nosocomial infection. N Engl J Med 1982;307:1562–6.

Weber DJ and Rutala WA. Environmental issues and nosocomial infections. In: Wenzel RP, editor. Prevention and control of nosocomial infection. 3rd ed. Baltimore (MD): Williams and Wilkins; 1997:491–514.

CHAPTER 10

Food

Johannes Oosterom, DVM, PhD

Key Issue: All people handling food should understand the sources and transmission routes of food-related pathogenic microorganisms and learn how to deal with food in a hygienic way, from production or collection until the final preparation and serving of meals.

Known Facts

- Meat and other food of animal origin are often contaminated with pathogenic microorganisms. However, fruits, vegetables, and cereals also may contain pathogenic microorganisms or toxins.
- Water can be contaminated through fecal pollution from man and animals. Fish, shellfish, and other food collected from polluted water may be contaminated.
- Consumption of contaminated food often leads to intestinal disease normally lasting a few days. However, in infants, diarrheal disease from contaminated food may be lethal.
- Contaminated food also can cause illnesses such as bovine tuberculosis, brucellosis, echinococcosis. Botulinum toxins may produce paralysis.

Controversial Issues: It is a misunderstanding that people should have regular exposure to food pathogens in order to increase and maintain their resistance. Particularly in infants and young children, gastrointestinal disease promotes the vicious and often lethal cycle of malnutrition and dehydration, growth retardation, and susceptibility to more infections. Every year, millions of infants die from intestinal disease.

Suggested Practice: The last and final line of defense against foodborne infectious disease is the preparation of food in the kitchen. Food handlers, including the people involved in food preparation at home, should be educated in general hygiene principles concerning food inspection, handling, storage, preparation, and serving.

Water should be collected from unpolluted sources and transported and stored hygienically.

General education on food hygiene should be placed into the framework of primary health care.

Several basic measures can eliminate pathogens in prepared food. Recommendations include: 1) thorough cooking of hazardous food, preferably immediately before consumption; 2) storage of prepared food either at low (<10°C) or high (>70°C) temperature; 3) protection from insects, rodents, and other animals; 4) reheating leftover food before consumption; 5) avoidance of cross-contamination during storage or preparation (usually from other raw food, hands, or contaminated equipment); 6) keeping the working environment (including equipment, working surfaces, and kitchen tools) clean; and 7) maintaining strict personal hygiene (particularly frequent handwashing).

Considerable efforts are needed to educate food handlers, managers of food establishments, kitchen workers, street vendors, and the general consumer. In developing countries, these efforts should be incorporated in the larger framework of primary health care.

Notwithstanding all these recommendations to prevent foodborne disease at the preparation level, food obtained from retail should have the lowest possible microbial contamination. This means that food processing should be done according to principles of Good Manufacturing Practices and the Hazard Analysis Critical Control Point (HACCP) system. National and international legislation should support this requirement.

References

Abdussalam M, Kaferstein FK. Food safety and primary health care. World Health Forum 1994;15:393–9.

Bryan FL. Risks of practices, procedures and processes that lead to outbreaks of foodborne diseases. J Food Protect 1988;51:663–73.

Oosterom J. Epidemiological studies and proposed preventive measures in the fight against human salmonellosis. Int J Food Microbiol 1991;12:41–52.

CHAPTER 11

WATER

M. Sigfrido Rangel-Frausto, MD, MSc

Key Issue: Because hospital water is not sterile, it can be a source for nosocomial infections.

Known Facts

- Hospital potable water should have <1 coliform bacterium/ 100 mL. High levels of bacteria in hospital water, dialysate water, sinks, faucets, and shower heads have been associated with disease outbreaks or hand colonization.
- Colonization of hospital water has been associated with cases of legionnaires' disease.
- Risk of illness may be influenced by several factors beside water contamination.

Suggested Practice

- High level of suspicion for cases of waterborne infections should be maintained, especially if clusters of infections occur.
- Hospital water should not be routinely cultured.
- Water used for dialysis should be sampled monthly and bacteria must be <200 bacteria/mL. Dialysate should be also cultured, and similar low levels of bacteria must be maintained.
- Use sterile water for rinsing nebulization devices and other semicritical respiratory-care equipment.
- Chloride levels in hospital water should be tested periodically.
- If possible, cooling towers should be placed away from hospital air-intake systems and designed such that the volume of aerosol drift is minimized. Install drift eliminators and regularly use an effective biocide, according to manufacturer's recommendations.
- Even one confirmed case of nosocomial legionnaires' disease requires an epidemiological and environmental investigation

for the source, including the water supply. Alert hospital personnel so that a high level of suspicion for the detection of new cases is maintained. This prospective surveillance should be maintained at least 2 months after the last case. If there is evidence of continuous transmission, hospital water should be sampled, and potential areas for aerosolized water should be looked for. If hospital water is contaminated with *Legionella* spp, start decontamination procedures:

1. **Superheating:** flushing outlet for at least 5 minutes with water >65°C, (post warning signs at each outlet being flushed to prevent scald injury), or
2. **Hyperchlorination:** >10 mg/L of free residual chlorine.
3. **Follow-up cultures** should be done at 2-week intervals for 3 months to evaluate actions taken.
   a. If no further positive cultures are found, collect monthly cultures for another 3 months.
   b. If positive cultures are found, reassess the implemented control measures, modify them accordingly, reimplement decontamination, and consider combination methods to decontaminate the water.

Table 11.1 Hospital Water-Linked Outbreaks

Microorganism	Reservoir	Infection
P. paucimobilis	Water bottles for rising tracheal suction	Pneumonia
S. marcescens	Water of humidifiers	Pneumonia
M. xenopi	Hot water taps	Pneumonia
M. chelonei	Contaminated equipment	Otitis
M. chelonei	Contaminated water tank	Nasal septum cellulitis
L. pneumophila	Hospital water, cooling towers	Pneumonia
Acinetobacter spp	Water bath used to thaw fresh plasma	Bacteremia
P. aeruginosa	Water bath used to thaw cryoprecipitate	Bacteremia
P. aeruginosa	Tub water contamination	Folliculitis, skin infections
C. difficile	Bath	Diarrhea

Summary: Many bacteria can survive in water and have been linked to nosocomial infections, including *Pseudomonas aeruginosa, Burkholderia cepacia, Serratia marcescens, Citrobacter freundii, Clostridium difficile, Acinetobacter baumani, Flavobacterium meningosepticum, Aeromonas hydrophila,* atypical mycobacteria, and *Legionella* spp, among others. Table 11.1 shows some examples of hospital water-linked outbreaks.

Routine cleaning, disinfection, and policies for use and changing of water from potential reservoirs should be implemented and periodically reviewed.

References

Centers for Disease Control and Prevention. Guideline for handwashing and hospital environmental control. Morb Mortal Wkly Rep 1985;37.

Centers for Disease Control and Prevention. Guideline for prevention of nosocomial pneumonia: Part 1. Issues on prevention of nosocomial pneumonia. Respir Care 1994;139:1191–236.

Weber DJ, Rutala WA. Environmental issues and nosocomial infections. In: Wenzel RP, editor. Prevention and control of nosocomial infections. 3rd ed. Baltimore (MD): Williams and Wilkins; 1997. p. 491–514.

CHAPTER 12

LABORATORY AREAS

Andreas Voss, MD, PhD, and Paul E. Verweij, MD, PhD

Key Issue: Laboratory workers are at occupational risk of exposure to microbiological pathogens that may cause inapparent to life-threatening infections. Laboratory-acquired infections are defined as all infections acquired through laboratory activities, regardless of their clinical/subclinical manifestations. Reviews of the incidence, consequences, and control of laboratory-acquired infections, such as that by Pike, have led to the development of laboratory safety programs. Despite these early guidelines, laboratory-acquired infections still occurred, probably due to a lack of instructions and/or poor compliance with safe laboratory practices. The emergence/re-emergence of HIV, Hantavirus, hepatitis C, and multiresistant *Mycobacterium tuberculosis* have not only renewed the interest in biosafety measurements but probably enhanced the compliance with these measures. Strategies for the prevention and management of laboratory-acquired infections should be aimed at containing biohazardous agents and educating laboratory workers about the occupational risks.

In general, biosafety programs include recommendations for work practices, laboratory design, personal protective equipment, and safety devices. Adherence to these biosafety guidelines can reduce the risk of exposure and consequent laboratory-acquired infections.

Known Facts
- During the 1980s, the most frequently found pathogens in a series of surveys were *Mycobacterium tuberculosis*, *Salmonella* spp, *Shigella* spp, hepatitis B virus, and hepatitis C virus.
- The annual incidence of laboratory-acquired infections is approximately 3/1000 employees in hospital laboratories.
- 43% (n = 162) of all laboratory-acquired infections are due

to *Rickettsia*, with *Coxiella burnetii* accounting for 95% of these infections.

- 75% of the viral infections were caused by arbo- and Hantaviruses.
- *Salmonella typhi*, *Brucella melitensis*, and *Chlamydia* spp were the most frequent causes of "bacterial" laboratory-acquired infections.

Exposure Resulting in Laboratory-Acquired Infection

Inhalation

- Mixing, vortexing, grinding, blending, and flaming a loop, may generate aerosols.
- In addition to airborne pathogens such as *M. tuberculosis*, airborne transmission in the laboratory may take place with organisms that do not naturally follow this route.

Ingestion

- Subconscious hand-to-mouth actions.
- Placing contaminated articles (e.g., pencils) or fingers (e.g., biting fingernails) in the mouth.
- Food consumption at the workplace or lack of hand disinfection before eating and smoking.
- 13% of all accidental laboratory-acquired infections are associated with mouth pipetting.

Inoculation

- Parenteral inoculation of infections materials through accidents with needles, blades, and broken glassware is one of the leading causes of laboratory-acquired infections.
- Needles and sharps used by laboratory workers (LWs) need to be disposed of in appropriate containers in order to reduce injury risk.

Contamination of Skin and Mucous Membranes

- Splashes onto the mucous membranes of the eyes, nasal cavity, and mouth, and hand-to-face actions may lead to transmission of pathogenic microorganisms.

- Handwashing and disinfection remain the major measures to prevent laboratory-acquired infections.

Biosafety Levels

In regard to the different groups/categories of laboratory-acquired infections, guidelines were developed that describe appropriate containment equipment, facilities, and procedures to be used by LWs. These guidelines are referred to as biosafety levels (BSLs). In general, four BSLs are described, which consist of combinations of primary and secondary barriers with microbiological practices. With Class 1 agents, hazards are minimal; Class 4 agents require maximal containment. Detailed information on BSLs recommended for specific bacterial, fungal, parasitic, and viral agents can be found in textbooks or the CDC website on Biosafety in Microbiological and Biomedical Laboratories at http://www.cdc.gov/od/ohs/biosfty/bmbl/section7.htm.

- BSL-1: lowest level of containment, microbiological safety, entirely based on standard laboratory practices. Recommended for work with microorganisms that are not known to cause infections in healthy adults, such as *Bacillus subtilis*.
- BSL-2: generally applied in bacteriology laboratories, during work with agents (e.g., *Salmonella* spp) associated with human disease of varying severity. When standard microbiological practices are applied, the agents may be handled on open benches, especially if primary barriers such as face protection, gowns, and gloves are used when appropriate. Consider use of BSCs and safety centrifuge.
- BSL-3: aimed at the containment of hazardous microorganisms primarily transmitted by aerosols, such as *Mycobacterium tuberculosis* or *Coxiella burnetii*. Use of stringent practices as well as primary and secondary safety equipment, including specific requirements for the facility, such

as a suitable ventilation system. All microorganisms of BSL-3 need to be processed in a biological safety cabinet (BSC).

- BSL-4: for agents causing life-threatening or untreatable diseases that can affect the laboratory worker via aerosols (e.g., hemorrhagic fever viruses). Manipulations are generally performed in a Class III BSC, or by personnel wearing full-body, air-supplied, positive-pressure suits. The facility itself is totally isolated from other laboratories and includes a specialized ventilation and waste management system.

Biosafety and Infection Control in the Microbiological Laboratory

Containment of hazardous agents is achieved by adherence to strict standard laboratory practices and techniques, supplemented by primary (safety equipment) and secondary barriers (facility design). Laboratory personnel need to be aware of potential hazards of infectious agents/materials. Practices and procedures to eliminate the risk of laboratory-acquired infections should be described in a laboratory manual.

Biological Safety Cabinets (BSCs) and Other Primary Barriers

- BSCs provide protection for personnel, the product, and the environment.
- Class I BSCs are negative pressured, ventilated, and are usually operated with an open front. They are designed for general microbiological research with low-to-moderate risk agents.
- Class II cabinets include HEPA-filtered vertical laminar airflow, providing protection from external contamination of the materials handled inside the BSC. Class IIA BSCs are used for microbiological procedures requiring biosafety level 2 or 3.
- Class III BSCs are totally enclosed cabinets with a gas-tight construction, providing the highest possible level of protection to the personnel and the environment, thereby suitable for work on biosafety level 3 or 4.

- Personal protection items, such as goggles, respirators, face shields, gloves, and gowns are frequently used in combination with BSCs.
- Additional equipment used to contain infectious splashes or aerosols are safety centrifuge cups, which prevent the release of infectious agents that can be transmitted during centrifugation.

Biosafety Practices

- Employ constant precautions in handling blood and body fluid, use/deposit sharps safely, and comply with hand disinfection (universal precautions).
- No eating, drinking, or smoking in the laboratory. Food may not be stored in refrigerators used for clinical specimens.
- No mouth pipetting—use proper mechanical devices.
- Decontaminate work surfaces daily and after spills.
- Provide well-fitting latex gloves to increase compliance with glove use.
- Face shields or masks and eye protection should be worn when splashing of blood or body fluids is possible.

Decontamination and Waste Disposal

- Tuberculocidal disinfectants should be used for regular decontamination of work surfaces and equipment.
- Use puncture-resistant, leak-proof containers for sharps.
- Separate potentially infectious waste and dispose in sturdy marked biohazard bags.

References

Grist NR, Emslie JAN. Infections in British clinical laboratories. J Clin Pathol 1991;44:667–9.

Harding L, Lieberman DF, Fleming DO, Richardson JH, Tulis JJ, Vesley D, editors. Laboratory safety: principles and practices. 2nd ed. Washington (DC): American Society for Microbiology; 1995. p. 7–15.

Jacobson JT, Orlob RB, Clayton JL. Infections acquired in clinical laboratories in Utah. J Clin Microbiol 1985;21:486-9.

Pike RM. Laboratory-associated infections: incidence, fatalities, causes and prevention. Ann Rev Microbiol 1979;33:41–66.

Sepkowitz KA. Occupational acquired infections in health care workers. Part I. Ann Intern Med 1996;125:826–4.

Sepkowitz KA. Occupational acquired infections in health care workers. Part II. Ann Intern Med 1996;125:917–28.

Sewell DL. Laboratory-acquired infections and biosafety. Clin Microbiol Rev 1995;8:389–405.

Sulkin SE, Pike RM. Laboratory-acquired infections. JAMA 1951;147:1740–5.

CHAPTER 13

THE PHARMACY

Mary D. Nettleman, MD, MS, and Meena H. Patel, MD

Key Issue: Medications must not become contaminated with pathogens during preparation or storage.

Known Facts: Infections have occurred when parenteral preparations have been improperly stored, handled, or have become significantly outdated.

Controversial Issues
- Infection control guidelines that govern the pharmacy also apply when medications are prepared on the wards or for home therapy.
- If medications are prepared outside of the pharmacy, it may be difficult to maintain asepsis.

Suggested Practice
- Employees should be trained in aseptic techniques before preparations.
- Written policies should be in place to describe the proper preparation and storage of medications.
- Employees should not prepare medications if they have active infections.
- Sterile medication should be prepared under aseptic conditions.
- Employees should wash hands thoroughly before handling medications.
- If storage containers are cracked or damaged, the solution should not be administered.
- Medications should be stored under conditions that meet manufacturers' guidelines.
- A tracking system should be devised in case of a product recall. The tracking system should allow identification of patients who received potentially contaminated medications.

Summary: Medications can become contaminated with bacteria, fungi, or viruses. Contamination can potentially occur through several routes, including

1. direct contact with human skin, contaminated surfaces, or syringes;
2. when medications are diluted with contaminated liquids; or
3. when airborne pathogens are allowed to contaminate solutions.

Each hospital pharmacy should develop policies for safe medication preparation and storage. Preparation of sterile medications may be done by technicians or nurses as well as pharmacists and sometimes may occur outside of the pharmacy. It is important that medications be safe from contamination regardless of where they are prepared or stored. Thus, policies should have input from all involved departments and disciplines. Written policies should also address education and training requirements and annual competency evaluation. As part of the competency evaluation, employees who prepare medications should be observed to ensure that they are following appropriate procedures. Policies should be reviewed annually to ensure that they still reflect current practices.

Products that are meant to be sterile, such as intravenous or intramuscular preparations, must be prepared under strict aseptic conditions. Many products arrive in a dehydrated form and must be reconstituted prior to use. It is vital that the liquid used to reconstitute the medication be sterile. Contaminants on the outside of the container must not be injected into the interior. If liquid is to be injected through a vial membrane, the membrane should be disinfected before being pierced. Syringes used to prepared medications should be sterile. Optimally, single-use, disposable syringes and needles should be used. In countries or settings where these products must be reused, they should be sterilized between uses.

Rooms in which medications are prepared should be free of visible dust, and traffic should be kept to a minimum. Surfaces should be clean. In general, medications should not be prepared in the same room that is used for unpacking supplies due to the risk of particulate matter in the air settling into solutions. Similarly, persons preparing sterile medications should wear clean clothing covers to minimize the amount of particles in the air.

Hands should be washed before and after medications are prepared. Sterile gloves are often required to maintain asepsis. Employees should not prepare any sterile products if they have rashes or broken skin on their hands. When preparing sterile or potentially toxic solutions, such as chemotherapies, laminar air flow hoods are strongly recommended.

Medications should be stored according to manufacturers' instructions. All medications should have an appropriate expiry date printed on the outside of the container. Environmental conditions should be checked periodically, including the temperature of refrigerators and the competency of laminar air flow hoods. Other equipment should be maintained according to the manufacturers' instructions.

In general, products that are stored for long periods before administration pose a greater risk than those that are prepared for immediate use. Multidose vials are at risk of contamination because they are entered again and again as the doses are removed. Strict attention to aseptic technique is necessary. All multidose products must be dated when opened.

As a quality control check, many pharmacies recommend testing a random sample of batches or solutions on a regular basis. Samples are passed through a submicron bacterial-retentive filter. The filter is then immersed in tryptic soy broth and incubated at 35°C for several days. If the broth becomes turbid, appropriate Gram's stains and subcultures are performed. Each hospital or pharmacy should have a means of tracking and retrieving contaminated products before they are administered and a means of identifying patients who have already received a contaminated product.

Although contaminated parenteral preparations have the highest potential for adverse events, oral preparations are also a concern. Ill patients may lack the normal gastric acid barrier or be greatly immunocompromised, thus making them susceptible to serious illness. In a situation analogous to food handlers, pharmacists and others who prepare oral medications might be able to transmit gastrointestinal pathogens to patients. Serious outbreaks have not been linked to oral medications but much of the potential risk can be eliminated by strict adherence to handwashing. Employees with active respiratory, gastrointestinal, or skin infections should not be permitted to handle medications.

In addition to infection control practices within the pharmacy, pharmacists should play a key role in the institutionwide infection control program. Antibiotic use and misuse are often at the root of outbreaks due to resistant pathogens. Sensible drug utilization requires the active participation of pharmacists.

References

American Society of Health-System Pharmacists. ASHP statement on the pharmacist's role in infection control. Am J Hosp Pharm 1986; 43:2006–8.

American Society of Hospital Pharmacists. ASHP technical assistance bulletin on quality assurance for pharmacy-prepared sterile products. Am J Hosp Pharm 1993;50:2386–98.

Santell JP, Kamalich RF. National survey of quality assurance activities for pharmacy-prepared sterile products in hospitals and home infusion facilities, 1995. Am J Health Syst Pharm 1996;53:2591–2605.

CHAPTER 14

OPERATING ROOM

Marie-Claude Roy, MD, MSc

Key Issue: The aim of keeping good infection control practices in the operating room (OR) is to decrease surgical site infections (SSIs), which represent an important proportion of nosocomial infections, with associated morbidity and excess health care costs. Modifying environmental factors associated with SSIs is an important area for infection control interventions.

Known Facts

- The majority of SSIs in the OR happen during the procedure. Few infections are acquired after the procedure if wounds are closed primarily. Therefore, shorter hospital stays and same-day surgery will not substantially decrease the incidence of SSI.

- Most SSIs arise from the patient's endogenous flora which contaminate the wound by direct contact. Therefore, the preoperative preparation of surgical patients should be meticulous to decrease the microbiologic burden of the patient's bowels, skin, respiratory tract, genital tract, etc., depending on the procedure being performed.

- Exogenous contamination of the wounds also is important, particularly to clean surgical procedures. Therefore, infection control practices in the operating theater deserve emphasis.

- The primary source of airborne bacteria in the OR is from the surgical team, who disperse many microorganisms from their skin, especially staphylococci.

Suggested Practice

Ventilation and Air Quality in the Operating Room.

- Optimally, operating rooms should be equipped with positive-pressure systems to ensure that air travels from ORs (aseptic zone) to adjacent areas (clean and protective zone).

- To remove airborne contaminants generated during surgery by patients or the surgical team in attendance, ventilation should filter air at a minimum of 20 changes/hour, of which at least four should be with fresh air.
- Keep the temperature of OR between 18°C and 24°C, with humidity of 50 to 55%.
- If the OR is not so equipped because of limited resources, focus on less expensive strategies to keep air as clean as possible: keep personnel to a minimum in the OR during a procedure, avoid excessive talking, keep doors and windows closed, and keep entries into the OR to a minimum during a procedure.

Preparation of the Patient in the OR.
- Avoid removing hair from the operative site unless it is so thick that it will interfere with the procedure.
- If hair removal is necessary, use clipping, or a depilatory instead of a razor. Surgical site infection rates increase 10-fold with the use of a razor when compared to a depilatory, clipping, or not removing hair.
- Removal of hair should be done immediately before surgeons perform the incision, not the night before surgery.
- Scrub the operative site with detergent, then apply an antiseptic soap, working from the proposed operative site outward.
- Antiseptics proposed for scrubbing include chlorhexidine, iodophors, and iodine.
- Sterile drapes should be applied after proper asepsis of the surgical site.
- If an antibiotic is prescribed for prophylaxis, ensure it is given less than 2 hours before the surgeon performs the incision, and ideally right before the procedure is begun. The risk of developing SSI increases two- to threefold if the antibiotic is given after the incision is performed, and more than sixfold if it is given too early (i.e., more than 2 hours before the incision). Therefore, antimicrobials should be given preferentially once the patient is in the OR.
- If a tourniquet is applied to the limb, as in orthopedic surgery, give the antibiotic at least 60 minutes before the incision.

Preparation of the Surgical Team.

- Wear a mask, headgear (which fully covers hair), and proper attire in the OR.
- Shoe covers can be replaced by ordinary shoes dedicated exclusively to the operating theater, as no differences exist in floor contamination whether personnel wear shoe covers or ordinary shoes (the former clearly costs more money to the hospital).
- Wear scrubs, which cover most bare skin, to decrease shedding of microorganisms from uncovered skin. People shed up to 10^9 epithelial cells per day, and many of these cells carry bacteria. The practice of wearing scrubs should be followed by all personnel working in the OR, not just those working in or near the operating field.
- Before the first procedure of the day, scrub arms and hands with chlorhexidine, iodophors, or hexachlorophene for at least 5 minutes, and for 2 to 5 minutes between subsequent procedures.
- Sterile gloves should be of good quality, as approximately 10% of gloves are inadvertently punctured during surgery.
- Two pairs of gloves should be worn in orthopedic surgery (where as many as 48% of gloves are punctured) and in other procedures with a high risk of bone fracture punctures (e.g., sternotomies).
- Good operative techniques clearly reduce the risk of SSI.
- Ensure that all equipment and surgical instruments necessary for the procedure are in the OR before the operation begins, thus reducing traffic and the need to open doors.

Controversial Issues.

- Patients should bathe or shower with an antiseptic before surgery. Although this practice reduces colonization of patient's skin with bacteria, it has not been proven to reduce colonization with *Staphylococcus aureus* in the nares, or reduce SSI rates.
- The use of brushes or sponges for preoperataive asepsis of hands and arms by surgeons and nurses can be replaced by

soap alone, as some studies demonstrated higher bacterial counts after brushing compared with the counts obtained after simple washing with soap. Significant savings may occur by not using sponges.

- Although cotton is not effective in reducing transfer of bacteria from the skin beneath the garment worn by surgical personnel to the surface of it, no other fabric has proven to reduce airborne contaminants in the OR while also providing comfort to the surgical team.
- The value of eradicating the patient carriage state of *Staphylococcus aureus* in the nares preoperatively with mupirocin is unproven.

The following practices do not reduce SSIs and should not be used:

- Having a transfer area where patients are transferred from ward trolleys to clean OR trolleys is expensive and has not proved cost effective in reducing floor contamination.
- Routinely culturing OR personnel is not necessary, unless an outbreak clearly links personnel to SSI cases. In this situation, and if *Staphylococcus aureus* is the cause of the outbreak, only culture the nares of implicated personnel, as this site has a 93% sensitivity.
- Routinely culturing the OR environment is also unnecessary, as inanimate objects and surfaces are seldom the cause of SSI. Settle plates used to evaluate airborne contaminants are not useful for the same reason.
- Using tacky mats.
- Scheduling dirty cases at the end of the day.

References

Gamer JS. CDC Guidelines for the prevention and control of nosocomial infections. Guideline for prevention of surgical wound infections, 1985. Am J Infect Control 1986;14:71–82.

Roy MC. The operating theater: a special environmental area. In: Wenzel RP, editor. Prevention and control of nosocomial infections. 3rd ed. Baltimore: Williams and Wilkins; 1997:515–38.

CHAPTER 15

EMERGENCY ROOM AND RECEIVING AREAS

Richard P. Wenzel, MD, MSc

Key Issue: Health care workers in emergency rooms and receiving areas need to protect themselves from bloodborne infections and also recognize and attempt to isolate quickly all patients with infections posing a risk to nearby personnel, patients, and visitors.

Known Facts: Universal precautions were promoted by the Centers for Disease Control and Prevention because of the inability to identify patients whose blood contained the hepatitis B or C virus, human immunodeficiency virus, and other pathogens. All blood should be considered potentially contaminated and efforts should be made to avoid direct contact, mucous membrane exposure, and sharps injuries.

Controversial Issues
- There is no controversy about the potential risk of transmission of blood disease to health care workers from patients.
- With respect to isolation, there are few data to show how effective various types of isolation are. Nevertheless, for most types of isolation precautions, the costs are low, and the rationale is based on available knowledge about the mode of transmission.
- No data exist to show how effective health care workers are at identifying patients at risk for transmitting infections.

Suggested Practice
- Careful handwashing before and after each patient encounter.
- Gloves should be worn when contact with blood and body fluids is likely.
- Goggles or face mask should be worn, if available, whenever splashing of blood or body fluids is likely.

- A triage person should be trained to identify patients with probable transmissible infections.
- Patients who appear unusually ill, especially with cough, should be isolated from other patients if possible.

Summary: Reasonable precautions as suggested above can minimize transmission of most infections in the emergency room i.e., those transmitted by close contact. There will still exist some risk of airborne diseases, such as those transmitted by droplet nuclei, especially influenza, measles, and tuberculosis. A room with an exhaust fan in the window will minimize airborne infections. Where this is not available, excellent ventilation will help.

References

Centers for Disease Control and Prevention Update: universal precautions for prevention of transmission of human immunodeficiency virus, hepatitis B virus, and other bloodborne pathogens in health care settings. Morb Mortal Wkly Rep 1988;37:377–82; 387–8.

Garner JS, Hierholzer WJ. Controversies in isolation policies and practices. In: Wenzel RP, editor. Prevention and control of nosocomial infections. 2nd ed. Baltimore: Williams and Wilkins; 1993. p. 70–81.

Centers for Disease Control and Prevention. Guidelines for preventing the transmission of tuberculosis in health care facilities. Morb Mortal Wkly Rep 1994;43(RR-130):1–132.

CHAPTER 16

HIV Infection and AIDS in Developing Countries

Philippe Van de Perre, MD, PhD,
Philippe Lepage, MD, PhD, and Jack Levy, MD PhD

Key Issue: Less than 15 years after it was first recognized in Africa, HIV infection is already the leading cause of adult deaths in many cities in developing countries, and has significantly increased childhood mortality. Despite considerable efforts to control the epidemic, HIV continues to spread at a rapid pace in developing countries. Out of an estimated 30 million people infected by HIV worldwide, 70% of the adults and 90% of the children are living in developing countries.

Known Facts

- Both HIV type 1 and HIV type 2 are circulating in developing countries; HIV-2 is less transmissible and less pathogenic than HIV-1.
- Both groups of HIV-1 (group M and group O) as well as all genotypic subtypes of HIV-1 group M (subtypes A to I) are found in developing countries. However, regional distribution of groups and subtypes varies considerably.
- Transfusion of HIV-contaminated blood is still responsible for about 10% of overall transmission events.
- Other types of bloodborne transmissions in medical settings are of lower public health importance.
- Sexual transmission remains by far the most frequent route of transmission in adults.
- Mother-to-child transmission of HIV involves almost exclusively HIV-1 and can occur in utero, during labor and delivery, and postnatally through breastfeeding. Mother-to-child transmission rate is estimated 20 to 30% in breastfeeding populations.
- Control of sexually transmitted diseases (STDs) at the com-

munity level is a cost-effective strategy to prevent sexual transmission of HIV.

- Blood banking organization, selection of blood donors, and HIV testing of blood donations are effective in preventing transfusion-associated infections.
- Prevention of mother-to-child transmission by treating HIV-infected pregnant women and their neonates with antiretrovirals is highly efficacious. In a clinical trial conducted in the US and France, a sophisticated regimen of zidovudine reduced mother-to-child transmission of HIV-1 by two-thirds. Recent evidence supports the efficacy of a shorter regimen of antiretrovirals. However, the efficacy of antiretrovirals when breastfeeding has to be continued (which is currently inevitable in many settings in developing countries) is unknown.
- More than 85% of fatal overwhelming infections associated with HIV as well as the first five causes of mortality in HIV-infected African patients are potentially amenable to a simple, effective, and frequently affordable anti-infectious treatment or prophylaxis. The most devastating public health impact of HIV-1 infection on other endemic diseases is on tuberculosis. In sub-Saharan Africa, the annual incidence of tuberculosis is more than 15-fold greater in HIV-infected individuals than in HIV-uninfected individuals.
- Clinical management of HIV-infected patients is largely based on access to nonspecific quality health care services for the diagnosis and treatment of opportunistic infections such as tuberculosis, pneumococcal disease, bacteremia, etc.

Controversial Issues

- What are the biological implications of HIV variability on transmission, pathogenesis, clinical expressions of disease, and response to treatment?
- What are the interactions between HIV infection and other tropical diseases (such as malaria, other parasitoses, malnutrition, etc.)?
- Are nonintravenous antiretroviral regimens and/or vitamin A

supplementation effective in reducing mother-to-child transmission of HIV? When should HIV-infected mothers breastfeed, and are there safe alternatives?

- What are the feasibility, efficacy, compliance, and long-term effects of prophylaxis of opportunistic infections such as TB with isoniazide, bacterial and protozoal infections with cotrimoxazole, or prevention of pneumococcal disease by vaccination?
- What is the role of antiretrovirals in the routine management of HIV infection in developing countries ?

Suggested Practice

- Prevention, clinical and psychosocial management, and fighting against discrimination/stigmatization are all integral parts of HIV/AIDS control programs. Each of these components is not sufficient in itself.
- These prevention strategies should be implemented:
  1. STD diagnosis and treatment at the community level (based on well-validated treatment algorithms);
  2. blood bank organization, blood donor selection, and HIV testing of blood donations;
  3. increase accessibility of mother and child to high quality health care services including prenatal care (prenatal clinics, basic obstetrical needs); and
  4. reinforce available health programs (TB control, malaria control, expanded program on immunization, maternal and child care, family planning, etc.).
- These psychosocial and clinical management strategies should be implemented:
  1. skilled, acceptable, accessible, and sustainable voluntary HIV counseling and testing services;
  2. simple clinical algorithms for clinical management of HIV disease and treatment of infectious episodes by means of available essential drugs and nutritional support;
  3. decentralized management and community support;
  4. new strategies to diagnose and treat TB (such as directly observed therapies); and

5. when possible, use of antiretrovirals, prophylaxis of opportunistic infections by antibiotics, and immunization against infections frequently associated with HIV.

References

Connor ED, Sperling RS, Gelber R, et al. Reduction of maternal-infant transmission of human immunodeficiency virus type 1 with ZDV treatment. N Engl J Med 1994;331:1173–80.

Grosskurth H, Mosha ., Todd J, et al. Impact of improved treatment of sexually transmitted diseases on HIV infection in rural Tanzania: randomised control trial. Lancet 1995;346:530–6.

Lucas SB, Hounnou A, Peacok C, et al. The mortality and pathology of HIV infection in a West African city. AIDS 1993;7:569–79.

TUBERCULOSIS

Gerd Fätkenheuer, MD

Key Issue: Tuberculosis is the leading cause of death from infectious diseases worldwide. Control of tuberculosis is a major public health issue, especially in developing countries.

Known Facts
- Identification and treatment of smear-positive cases are crucial for tuberculosis control.
- A high percentage of patients with tuberculosis are coinfected with HIV.
- Directly observed therapy (DOT) improves the outcome of tuberculosis in HIV-negative persons as well as in HIV-positive persons.
- Multidrug-resistant tuberculosis (MDR-TB) dramatically increases the mortality of tuberculosis.
- Poor adherence to antituberculous therapy is the major risk factor for MDR-TB and for poor outcome of therapy.
- Chemoprophylaxis can reduce morbidity from tuberculosis in HIV-infected persons with positive skin test.
- Vaccination with bacille Calmette-Guérin (BCG) may reduce the risk of tuberculosis. Most data support its use in high prevalence areas only for children, primarily to prevent TB meningitis.

Controversial Issues: Chemoprophylaxis of children and of tuberculin skin test-negative HIV-infected persons has not proven to be cost effective in developing countries.

- The necessity of follow-up smear examinations in resource-poor countries is an issue of debate.
- HIV-infected persons with tuberculosis have been supposed to be less infective than HIV-negative patients due to a high-

er rate of smear-negative cases. However, many studies have documented the spread of TB from persons coinfected with HIV.

Suggested Practice:
- Perform a vigorous diagnostic workup for TB (including smears and chest X-ray) in any patient with respiratory symptoms.
- Separate patients with suspected TB and with confirmed TB from other patients in the hospital.
- Perform DOT short course in an ambulatory setting.
- Vaccinate children with BCG in high prevalence areas.

Summary: Tuberculosis has been one of the major killers in the history of mankind. While in developed countries incidence rates declined dramatically within the last decades due to improvement of socioeconomic conditions, in developing countries the burden of disease is increasing. According to estimates by the World Health Organization (WHO), 90 million new tuberculosis cases will occur during the 1990s causing 30 million TB-related deaths, and 95% of these will be in developing countries. Up to 40% of patients with tuberculosis will be coinfected with HIV, and tuberculosis is the single most common cause of death in HIV-infected Africans.

Since most cases of tuberculosis are transmitted by smear-positive patients, identification of these persons and consequent treatment with combination chemotherapy remains the cornerstone of tuberculosis control. Microscopic examination of three sputum samples (Ziehl-Neelsen stain) is the standard procedure to rule out active pulmonary tuberculosis. A certain percentage of smear-negative patients (especially HIV-infected persons) may have positive cultures but cultures are not routinely performed in developing countries due to lack of resources and high costs.

Combination chemotherapy has to be initiated in each patient with proven or clinically suspected tuberculosis. Three principles are essential for the management of patients with tuberculosis: use at least two potent drugs, maintain treatment over an extended period, and ensure regular administration of medication. Isoniazid, rifampin, pyrazinamide, and ethambutol are the drugs of choice. Thiocetazone frequently causes severe side effects in HIV-infected patients and should not be used in them. With all drug regimens, adherence to and completion of therapy are crucial for avoidance of drug resistance and for the achievement of definite cure. Directly observed therapy (DOT) can substantially improve the outcome of antituberculous therapy and is now promoted by the WHO. Intermittent administration of DOT (Table 17.1) reduces costs, can be given on an ambulatory basis, and may be supervised by volunteers.

For economic reasons and for prevention of nosocomial transmission of tuberculosis, hospitalization should be restricted to severely ill patients. Standard requirements for hospitalized patients in developed countries include isolation in private rooms with negative air pressure and the use of approved masks. These measures are usually not available in developing countries.

Table 17.1 Proposed Regimens for Short-Course, Ambulatory, Intermittent, Directly Observed Therapy of Tuberculosis

1	INH + RMP + PZA + EMB (3 doses weekly for 6 months)
2	INH + RMP + PZA (daily for 2 months); followed by: INH + RMP (2 doses weekly for 4 months)
3	INH + RMP + PZA + EMB (3 doses weekly for 2 months); followed by: INH + RMP (3 doses weekly for 4 months)
4	INH + RMP + PZA + EMB (daily for 2 weeks); followed by: INH + RMP + PZA + EMB (2 doses weekly for 6 weeks); followed by: INH + RMP (2 doses weekly for 16 weeks)

INH = isoniazid; RMP = rifampin; PZA = pyrazinamide; EMB = ethambutol

Preventive therapy of children under 5 years old with household contact to tuberculosis cases has been advocated by the WHO. Prophylaxis with isoniazid for 6 months or with multidrug regimens containing isoniazid and rifampin for 3 months have been shown to be efficacious in both non-HIV-infected persons and HIV-infected persons with positive skin reaction to purified protein derivative (PPD). However, whether preventive therapy on a large scale is feasible and cost effective in developing countries has still to be examined.

Vaccination is another tool of tuberculosis control. It is estimated that 80% of individuals are vaccinated with BCG worldwide. BCG vaccination provides a good protection of dissemination and lethal complications in children and is therefore indicated in regions with a high prevalence of tuberculosis.

References

De Cock KM, Wilkinson D. Tuberculosis control in resource-poor countries: alternative approaches in the era of HIV [comments]. Lancet 1995;346:675–7.

Porter JD. Mycobacteriosis and HIV infection: the new public health challenge. J Antimicrob Chemother 1996;37:113–20.

Raviglione MC, Snider DE Jr, Kochi A. Global epidemiology of tuberculosis. Morbidity and mortality of a worldwide epidemic. JAMA 1995;273:220–6.

Whalen CC, Johnson JL, Okwera A, et al. A trial of three regimens to prevent tuberculosis in Ugandan adults infected with the human immunodeficiency virus. Uganda-Case Western Reserve University Research Collaboration. N Engl J Med 1997;337:801–8.

Wilkinson D, Davies GR, Connolly C. Directly observed therapy for tuberculosis in rural South Africa, 1991 through 1994 [comments]. Am J Public Health 1996;86:1094–7.

CHAPTER 18

DIARRHEA

Made Sutjita, MD, and Herbert L. DuPont, MD

Key Issues: A diarrheal disease outbreak in health care facilities may affect patients, health care workers, and visitors. Recognizing these risk factors, surveillance, and initiation of prompt infection control management practices will reduce the morbidity and mortality rate.

Known Facts

- Microorganisms that cause infectious diarrhea outbreaks in the community are also able to cause a nosocomial outbreak in hospitalized patients. However, some forms of diarrheal disease, such as food poisoning caused by *Bacillus cereus*, *Clostridium botulinum*, and *Staphylococcus aureus*, have not been demonstrated to be directly transmissible from person to person in the hospital.

- Common bacteria reported to cause nosocomial gastroenteritis include various strains of diarrheagenic *E. coli*, *Salmonella* spp, *Shigella* spp, *Y. enterocolitica*, *Vibrio cholerae* and *C. difficile*. Viral agents such as rotavirus, Norwalk virus, and adenovirus have been implicated in nosocomial outbreaks. In a childcare setting, enteroviruses, such as polioviruses, have the potential to cause an outbreak in a nonimmune population as do *Giardia lamblia* and the conventional enteropathogens.

- It is important to distinguish between nosocomial diarrhea and infectious nosocomial gastroenteritis. Nosocomial diarrhea or diarrhea of noninfectious origin, such as that caused by cathartics, tube feeding, inflammatory bowel disease, surgical resection, and anastomoses, should be differentiated from diarrhea of infectious origin.

- The rate of nosocomial gastroenteritis varies among hospitals and services. The NNIS (National Nosocomial Infections Surveillance) in the USA reported a nosocomial gastroenteritis infection rate of 2.27 per 1000 discharged, for the period January 1990 through December 1994. Infection rates of nosocomial gastroenteritis in developing countries is not exactly known. Nonetheless, outbreaks of nosocomial gastroenteritis are being reported with increasing frequency. *Salmonella* spp are the most common cause of nosocomial gastroenteritis in India, Pakistan, and Tunisia.

- Risk factors for nosocomial gastroenteritis can be classified by intrinsic and extrinsic factors. Intrinsic factors include abnormality in the mucosal defense, such as achlorhydria, impairment of intestinal motility, and alteration of normal enteric flora. Neonates with undeveloped immunity or patients with an immune deficiency state, such as those on immunosuppressive drugs or with AIDS, are at an increased risk to develop nosocomial gastroenteritis. Extrinsic factors include nasogastric tube feeding while receiving cimetidine, which allows intestinal colonization of bacteria. Such a setting is normally found in an intensive care unit.

- Modes of transmission of infectious agents causing gastroenteritis are typically through the fecal-oral route. The transmission occurs either by contact spread from patient to patient, patient to health care worker (HCW), or HCW to patient (either direct or indirect), or through common-vehicle spread. Contaminated vehicles such as food, water, medications, or devices and equipment can play a significant role in the transmission of the agents.

- Definitions of diarrhea vary but generally include the passage of liquid or watery stools, three or more times per day. Microorganisms that invade the intestinal mucosa often elicit a febrile response in addition to causing diarrhea. Diarrhea in a patient with unexplained fever should be diagnosed as infectious gastroenteritis regardless of culture results. If a patient is febrile or diarrhea occurs in a patient whose fever has other likely causes, the identification of pathogenic microorganisms is necessary to establish the diagnosis.

- The usual known incubation period of an infectious agent is important in determining whether a given infection is nosocomial. The interval between the time of admission and the onset of clinical symptoms must be longer than the known minimum incubation period of the infectious agent. Alternatively, nosocomial gastroenteritis can be determined if a stool culture obtained shortly before or just after admission is negative for a given pathogenic agent and the agent is subsequently cultured from the patient's stool.

Controversial Issues

- *Salmonella* spp were reported as the most common cause of nosocomial gastroenteritis in some developing countries but the infection rate of other enteric pathogens is not well known. Without the established mechanism for routinely reporting nosocomial outbreaks, the "true" infection rate of given pathogens is underestimated.
- The availability of "over-the-counter" antibiotics without a physician prescription in many developing regions may lead to the development of resistant microorganisms. This often complicates the management of a diarrheal disease outbreak.

Suggested Practice

- Effective handwashing is among the most important measures to reduce the risks of transmitting microorganisms from one person to another or from one site to another in the same patient.
- Gloves play an important role in reducing the risk of microorganism transmission, and prevent contamination of the hands when touching patients and fomites. Attempts should be made to reduce the likelihood of the hands of the HCW being contaminated with microorganisms from a patient or a fomite and of infecting another patient. In this case, gloves must be changed between patient contacts and hands must be washed after gloves are removed.

- Gowns and other protective apparel provide barrier protection and reduce the transmission of microorganisms. Gowns, boots, or shoe covers provide greater protection to the skin when splashes or large quantities of infective material are present or anticipated. When a gown is worn during the care of a patient infected with an epidemiologically important microorganism, it should be removed before leaving the patient's environment.

- A private room is important to prevent direct or indirect contact transmission of the microorganism. Whenever possible, a patient with infectious diarrhea is placed in a private room with handwashing and toilet facilities. A sign of "contact isolation" should be placed in front of the door to warn visitors or other HCWs. Patients infected by the same microorganism may share a room (cohorting), provided they are not infected with another potentially transmissible microorganism.

- Limiting the transport of a hospitalized patient with infectious diarrhea may also reduce the opportunities for transmission of the microorganism in the hospital.

- The patient's room, bed, and bedside equipment should be cleaned thoroughly. In a patient with stool positive for VRE, adequate disinfection of environmental surfaces, i.e., bed rails, tables, carts, commodes, doorknobs, or faucet handles, is indicated. Enterococci are known to survive in the inanimate environment for prolonged periods of time.

- Urine, feces, and soiled linen should be considered potentially infectious and handled or disposed of appropriately as discussed elsewhere. Personnel handling these materials should wear gloves and other protective apparel as described above.

Summary: It is important to establish a hospital surveillance program in which clinical patterns of infection are monitored on a regular basis. A "low-budget" surveillance program probably can be carried out by daily review and tabulation of bacteriologic reports from the hospital microbiology laboratory. Cooperation and effective communication between hospital epidemiology and microbiology laboratory personnel is essential.

In addition to the patient population, surveillance must include hospital personnel, particularly food handlers, nurses, and medical staff. An employee health service or an employee clinic ideally should be easily accessible to each employee. Food handlers, nurses, and ancillary staff having direct contact with patients should report to the employee health service when they experience an episode of diarrhea. In this case, stool cultures should be performed and the ill employee temporarily removed from work until the clinical course of the disease and culture result can be evaluated. Workers should not return to work until their diarrhea is resolved and two stool cultures obtained at least 24 hours apart show negative results.

A nosocomial infectious gastroenteritis outbreak may occur due to the transmission from carriers of a specific pathogenic microorganism. Carriers can be patients or hospital personnel. Surveillance carried out on a regular basis should detect any episodes of gastroenteritis among patients and hospital personnel. Temporal clustering of cases should alert infection control personnel to the possibility of an outbreak. Occasionally, an outbreak may occur due to a contaminated vehicle such as food, equipment, or oral medication. If such a vehicle is identified, its removal or disinfection may help to terminate the outbreak.

Patients with infectious gastroenteritis should be discharged from the hospital as soon as their condition allows them to be managed on an outpatient basis.

References

Cookson ST, Hughes JM, and Jarvis WR. Nosocomial gastrointestinal infections. In: Wenzel RP, editor. Prevention and control of nosocomial infections. 3rd ed. Baltimore: Williams & Wilkins; 1997. p. 925–75.

DuPont HL, Ribner BS. Infectious gastroenteritis. In: Bennett JV, Brachman PS, editors. Hospital infections. 4th ed. Philadelphia: Lippincott-Raven; 1998. p. 537–50.

Slutsker L, Villarino ME, Jarvis WR, Goulding J. In: Bennett JV, Brachman PS, editors. Hospital infections. 4th ed. Philadelphia: Lippincott-Raven; 1998. p. 333–41.

Weinstein JW, Hierholzer W Jr, Garner JS. Isolation precautions in hospitals. In: Bennett JV, Brachman PS, editors. Hospital infections. 4th ed. Philadelphia: Lippincott-Raven; 1998. p. 189–98.

CHAPTER 19

SKIN AND SOFT TISSUE INFECTIONS

Antoni Trilla, MD, MSc

Key Issue: Skin and soft tissue (SST) infections are not uncommon in the hospital setting. In addition to localized complications, skin and soft tissue infections may cause life-threatening bacteremias or sepsis.

Known Facts: The most common causative agent is *Staphylococcus aureus*, followed by *Streptococcus pyogenes* and anaerobic gram-negative bacilli. In special populations (diabetic patients, burn wounds), aerobic gram-negative bacilli, including *Pseudomonas aeruginosa*, should also be considered.

Staphylococcus aureus is found over the normal skin, as a transient organism, often linked to nasal carriage (anterior nares). Pre-existing conditions, such as tissue injuries (surgical wounds, trauma, pressure sores) or skin inflammation (dermatitis), and other systemic diseases (insulin-dependent diabetes, cancer, chronic renal failure on hemodialysis, intravenous drug abuse, and infection with HIV) are well-known risk factors for skin colonization and/or secondary infection by *Staphylococcus aureus*.

Staphylococcal Skin Infections

Key Issue: Impetigo is the most common skin infection. It is a superficial primary skin infection, most often caused by *Streptococcus pyogenes* infection (90%) or *Staphylococcus aureus* (10%). Impetigo may appear as a complication of other skin disorders, like eczema, varicella, or scabies.

Known Facts: Often seen in children, impetigo is readily transmitted in households and hospitals. When considering the diagnosis of impetigo, one should remember the increasing frequency of skin disorders in HIV-infected patients.

Suggested Practice: Standard hygienic measures and contact isolation procedures should be used in patients with impetigo. This practice must be encouraged especially in neonatal and pediatric intensive care units, as well as for patients with rashes or HIV.

Controversial Issues: The use of several antibiotics (mupirocin, fusidic acid, erythromycin, tetracycline) as topical treatment for impetigo had been shown to have ~90% efficacy in clinical trials. The use of topical antibiotics decreases bacterial colonization and infection and promotes faster wound healing. Oral antibiotic treatment (erythromycin, antistaphylococcal penicillin, amoxicillin + clavulanic acid) has also been used with a similar success rate. However, the emergence of multidrug-resistant *S. aureus* strains, including methicillin-resistant *S. aureus* (MRSA) and mupirocin-resistant strains, is a matter of concern and should be closely monitored when topical treatments with special agents like mupirocin are used for long periods of time.

Staphylococcal Scalded Skin Syndrome (SSSS)

Key Issue: SSSS is a severe *Staphylococcus aureus* infection with extensive bullae and exfoliation.

Known Facts: It usually occurs in children, and rarely in adults. Several epidemics have been reported in nurseries and neonatal intensive care units (NICU). The clinical picture is related to the production of a powerful exotoxin by the *S. aureus* strains. Most cases present with acute fever and a scarlatiniform skin rash. Large bullae soon appear, followed by exfoliation. Also known as toxic epidermal necrolysis, this syndrome can be caused by other infections or drug reactions.

Suggested Practice: The use of an antistaphylococcal penicillin is the preferred initial antibiotic treatment. Topical treatment consists of cool saline compresses.

Controversial Issues: The use of corticosteroids alone is not recommended for SSSS.

Skin and Soft Tissue Infections in Diabetic Patients

Key Issue: Diabetic patients are at higher risk for developing skin and soft tissue (SST) infections from *Staphylococcus aureus*.

Known Facts: Hyperglycemic states are linked with higher nasal and skin carriage of *S. aureus* strains. The impaired cell-mediated immunity of these patients is another important factor.

Controversial Issues: Diabetic patients may present with a variety of clinical syndromes due to SST infections. One severe condition is the acute dermal gangrene syndrome. This syndrome, related to more deep tissue infection and dermal necrosis, is often associated with prior trauma or surgery. It includes two different conditions:

1. Necrotizing fasciitis, affecting the fascia and producing complete necrosis of subcutaneous tissue. This syndrome is often associated with high fevers, sepsis, septic shock, and a high mortality rate (30%).
2. Progressive bacterial gangrene, a more slowly progressive infection, usually related to surgical wounds, ileostomy sites, and exit site of drains (intra-abdominal or thoracic due to empyema), which affects the upper third of the hypodermis. The patient usually has a low grade or no fever, and local signs of infection are predominant.

Other syndromes include Meleney's gangrene, when the clinical picture is slowly progressive and without deep fascial involvement, Fournier's gangrene, if the perineal zone is involved, streptococcal gangrene, if *Streptococcus pyogenes* is the causative agent, or nonclostridial anaerobic synergistic myonecrosis when the muscle is also involved. These SST disorders are nearly always due to polymicrobial infections, with

Streptococcus pyogenes and *Staphylococcus aureus* commonly isolated.

Suggested Practice: Systemic antimicrobial treatment based on likely pathogens (including penicillin, antistaphylococcal penicillin, amoxicillin + clavulanic acid, a first- or second-generation cephalosporin) together with extensive and repeated surgical débridement are always needed and must be started early.

Burn Wound Infections

Key Issue: Burn wound patients and burn wound units are potential portals of entry for nosocomial outbreaks of MRSA and *Pseudomonas aeruginosa*. *Staphylococcus aureus* is responsible for 25% of all burn wound infections, followed by *P. aeruginosa*.

Known Facts: The most likely reservoirs for these infections are the hands and nares of health care workers (*S. aureus*, MRSA), the burn wound itself and the GI tract of burn patients (*S. aureus, P. aeruginosa*), and the inanimate environment of the burn unit, including the surfaces and/or the equipment (*S. aureus*, MRSA, *P. aeruginosa*).

Suggested Practice: Common standard isolation precautions, together with contact isolation precautions are important to prevent nosocomial infections in burn units and patients. Topical treatment using mafenide acetate, silver sulfadiazine, bacitracin/ neomycin/polymyxin, 2% mupirocin, together with systemic, antistaphylococcal and anti-*Pseudomonas* antibiotics should be reserved for documented or clinical infections.

Pressure Sores (Decubitus Ulcers)

Key Issue: Pressure sores appear in 6% of patients admitted to health care institutions (range 3 to 17%), and are the leading cause of infection in long-term care facilities.

Known Facts: The prevention of pressure sores includes the control of local factors such as unrelieved pressure, friction, moisture, or systemic factors such as low serum albumin, fecal incontinence, and poor hygienic measures. The infection is polymicrobial, and includes gram-negative bacilli, *Staphylococcus aureus*, *Enterococcus* spp and anaerobes. The average number of isolates in infected pressure sores is four, including three aerobic and one anaerobic bacteria. Pressure sores are sometimes associated with severe systemic complications, including bacteremia, septic thrombophlebitis, cellulitis, deep-tissue and fascial necrosis, and osteomyelitis. The development of clinical tetanus is unlikely, although still possible. In patients with bacteremia and pressure sores, the sores were considered to be the source of the bacteremia in half the cases. Overall mortality was 55%, with approximately 25% of deaths attributable to the infection. Therefore, pressure sores must be considered a potential source for nosocomial bacteremia.

Suggested Practice: Antibiotic treatment, together with surgical care and débridement of the sores, is needed. Taking into account the most likely microorganisms, a second-generation cephalosporin is one of the drugs of choice. The combination of a beta-lactam antibiotic with an aminoglycoside, or clindamycin plus an aminoglycoside, or a cephalosporin plus metronidazole are other good therapeutic options.

Nosocomial Bacteremia Due to SST Infection

Key Issue: Nosocomial bacteremia secondary to SST infections has a low frequency rate. According to National Nosocomial Infections Surveillance (NNIS) data, only 5 to 8% of all bacteremic episodes were secondary to SST infections. In Spain, different serial prevalence surveys identified that the national rate of nosocomial bacteremia related to SST infections was 5.3 to 6.6%.

Known Facts: Patients with poorly controlled diabetes and cancer are a high-risk group for developing this infection. In one large series from the US National Cancer Institute, 12% of all bacteremic episodes in cancer patients were secondary to SST infection. However, only 6% of those cases were associated with severe neutropenia. In neutropenic patients, ecthyma gangrenosum due to *Pseudomonas aeruginosa* SST infection must be always considered. Intravenous drug abuse (IVDA), involving heroin, heroin plus cocaine, or heroin plus other drugs, is a worldwide problem. SST infections are common among IVD abusers, ranging from 6 to 8% of all infections in a large Spanish study. *S. aureus* is the most common microorganism (one-third of cases). The common clinical presentations are subcutaneous abscesses, cellulitis, and lymphangitis, most often (60%) located in upper extremities. Bacteremia is one of the most severe and common complications among IVD abusers, with 40% of all episodes due to *S. aureus*.

Suggested Practice: If bacteremia develops in an IVD abuser, septic thrombophlebitis or endocarditis should be considered, and antibiotic treatment started as soon as possible.

References

Trilla A, Miro JM. Identifying high risk patients for *Staphylococcus aureus* infections: skin and soft tissue infections. J Chemother 1995;7:27–33.

Johnston C. Diabetic skin and soft tissue infections. Curr Opin Infect Dis 1994;7:214–8.

Bryan CS, Dew CE, Reynolds KL. Bacteremia associated with decubitus ulcers. Arch Intern Med 1983;143:2093–5.

Vaque J, Rossell U J, Trilla A et al. Nosocomial infections in Spain: results of five serial prevalence surveys. Infect Control Hosp Epidemiol 1996;17:293–7.

CHAPTER 20

BLOODSTREAM INFECTIONS

Didier Pittet, MD, MS, and Stephan Harbarth, MD

Key Issue: Most nosocomial bloodstream infections (BSIs) are related to the use of an intravascular device. Bloodstream infection rates are substantially higher among patients with intravascular devices than those without such devices. Appropriate care of intravascular devices prevents infection.

Known Facts: The crude mortality of nosocomial BSI is high (25 to 60%), and the attributable mortality averages 25%. In the USA, nosocomial BSI causes as many as 3.5 million additional hospital days per year, accounting for 3.5 billion dollars in costs related to excess stay. Nosocomial bloodstream infections have been divided into two categories:

- Primary bloodstream infections which occur without any recognizable focus of infection with the same organism at another anatomic site at the time of positive blood culture. Episodes of bloodstream infections secondary to intravenous or arterial lines are typically classified as primary BSI (CDC definitions).
- Secondary bloodstream infections which develop subsequent to a documented infection with the same microorganism at another body site

Intravascular devices are responsible for at least a third of all primary BSIs and a variety of local or systemic infectious complications.

The species of microorganisms causing BSI changed in the last 2 decades. The proportion of primary bacteremias caused by coagulase-negative staphylococci and enterococci more than doubled, and *Candida* spp appeared in the list of the ten leading pathogens. Whereas *Escherichia coli* and *Klebsiella pneumoniae* together with *Staphylococcus aureus* were the three leading pathogens in the mid-1970s, the former two caused only 10% of all episodes of nosocomial bacteremia both in 1983 and 1986–1989. Coagulase-negative staphylococci currently account for one-fourth of BSIs. In the past, coagulase-negative staphylococci frequently were considered contaminants. However, recent studies have shown that only a single blood culture positive for coagulase-negative staphylococci is sometimes associated with clinically relevant episodes of bloodstream infection. Thus, each episode of coagulase-negative staphylococci bacteremia mandates careful consideration.

Controversial Issues: The following are practices for which insufficient evidence or consensus regarding efficacy exists:

- Use of impregnated or coated intravascular catheters or needleless intravascular devices
- Frequency of replacement of IV tubing used for intermittent infusions and frequency of routine replacements of dressings used on catheter sites
- Routine use of heparin or cortisone in parenteral solutions to reduce risk of phlebitis

Suggested Practice: Prevention of device-related BSIs includes the following recommended practices:

- Education and training of health care workers
- Surveillance for catheter-related BSIs
- Handwashing
- Barrier precautions during catheter insertion (sterile gloves, gowns) and maximal barrier precautions (sterile gloves, gowns, masks, large drape) in neutropenic and high-risk patients
- Catheter-site care (cutaneous antisepsis, avoidance of moisture accumulation, sterile dressing)
- Removal of catheter as soon as clinically indicated
- Immediate replacement of tubings used to administer blood, blood products, or lipid emulsions

- Cleaning injection ports with 70% alcohol before use
- Quality control of intravenous admixtures
- No routine use of filters for infection control purposes
- Designated trained IV teams
- For central venous catheters, using subclavian, rather than jugular insertion sites
- No routine replacement of central venous catheters in a regular time period
- No guidewire-assisted catheter exchange in case of infection
- Subcutaneous tunnelized catheters for long-term use in high-risk patients

Summary: Important findings concerning the prevention of catheter-related bloodstream infections include moisture accumulation under transparent semipermeable dressings and placement in the internal jugular vein. The risk of infection has been reduced by the use of maximal sterile barriers (gloves, gown, mask, large drape) for catheter insertions, by the use of alcoholic preparations of chlorhexidine to disinfect the skin at the insertion site, and subcutaneous tunnelization of the central venous catheter. The use of coated catheters has been associated with lower infection rates and may be recommended for certain categories of patients in the near future.

References

Maki DG, Mermel LA. Infections due to infusion therapy. In: Bennett J, Brachman P, editors. Nosocomial infections. 4th ed. 1998. p. 689–739.

Pearson ML and the Hospital Infection Control Practices Advisory Committee. Guideline for prevention of intravascular device-related infections. Infect Control Hosp Epidemiol 1996;17:438–73.

Pittet D. Nosocomial bloodstream infections. In: Wenzel RP, editor. Prevention and control of nosocomial infections. 3rd ed. Baltimore: Williams & Wilkins; 1997 p. 712–69.

CHAPTER 21

HOSPITAL-ACQUIRED URINARY TRACT INFECTIONS

Slavko Schönwald, MD, PhD, and Bruno Baršić, MD

Key Issue: Hospital-acquired urinary tract infections (HUTI) are the most common hospital-acquired infections, accounting for about 40% of the total number of all nosocomial infections. About 80% of all HUTI are associated with urinary catheters, followed by other urogenital instrumentation. Their incidence can be significantly reduced by applying recommendations for prevention of catheter-associated urinary tract infections.

Known Facts

- Hospital-acquired urinary tract infections are caused by a variety of pathogens, many of which, such as *Escherichia coli*, *Klebsiella* spp, *Proteus* spp, *Enterococcus* spp, *Enterobacter* spp are part of the patient's endogenous bowel flora.
- The isolation of pathogens such as *Serratia marcescens* and *Pseudomonas cepacia* have special epidemiologic significance and indicate in the majority of cases acquisition from an exogenous source.
- Numerous studies have shown that an increase in infection rates is associated with unjustified long-term catheter use. The period of catheterization should be as short as medically possible to minimize the risk of infection.
- The most common reasons for entry of bacteria into the bladder during catheterization:
  - poor aseptic preparation at the time when the catheter is inserted
  - disconnection of the catheter and drainage tube
  - contamination during irrigation
  - colonization of the drainage bag and retrograde flow of contaminated urine into the bladder

Controversial Issues

- In selected groups of patients, use of condom catheter drainage systems decreases the risk of HUTI but in some patients (e.g., agitated patients), their use has been associated with increased risk of HUTI.
- Use of a suprapubic catheter decreases the risk of HUTI. This practice has not been proven by controlled clinical studies.
- Intermittent catheterization decreases the risk of HUTI. This practice has not been proven by controlled clinical studies.
- Routine bacteriologic monitoring of catheterized patients to detect new HUTI. Its potential benefit has not been adequately investigated. Finding of transient bacteriuria can lead to unnecessary antibiotic use.

The efficacy of prophylactic systemic antibiotics to prevent HUTI is transient and associated with the selection of antibiotic-resistant microorganisms.

Suggested Practice

- Educate personnel in correct techniques of catheter insertion and care.
- Catheterize only when necessary.
- Emphasize handwashing.
- Insert catheter using aseptic technique and sterile equipment.
- Secure catheter properly.
- Maintain closed sterile drainage continuously.
- Obtain urine samples aseptically.
- Maintain unobstructed urine flow.
- Avoid irrigation unless needed to prevent or relieve obstruction.

Summary: Urinary catheterization is a precondition for the onset of the majority of nosocomial urinary tract infections. Catheter-associated urinary tract infections are generally assumed to be benign, and in some cases the infection resolves with the removal of the catheter. However, HUTI can lead to bacteremia. It has been estimated that 18 to 25% of hospital bacteremias are related to HUTI. Hospital-acquired urinary tract infections may occur not only sporadically but also in smaller and larger epidemics, where they are most frequently caused by multiresistant pathogens.

A continuously closed drainage system is the cornerstone of infection control. With an open urinary drainage system, urinary infection often occurs after 3 to 4 days. Errors in maintaining sterile closed drainage also predispose patients to infection. In closed urinary drainage systems, the risk of infection may be reduced by proper catheter insertion and the reduction of unnecessary manipulation of the catheter after insertion. Infection usually occurs when the microorganisms adhere to the urethral epithelial cells and proliferate around the urethral meatus with retrograde entry into the bladder. It is important to maintain the cleanness of the periurethral area to prevent colonization and its consequences. Other preventive measures to block the entry of bacteria into the space between catheter outer surface and urethra failed. However, the best method for prevention of HUTI is avoiding the use of an indwelling catheter, whenever possible (Table 21.1).

When urinary catheterization is necessary the time of catheter use should be reduced to a minimum. Manipulation of catheter should be done only by hospital staff, family members, and patients themselves who know the correct technique of aseptic insertion and maintenance of the catheter.

Additional measures which may be helpful in reducing HUTI include the periodical re-education of personnel involved in catheter care, use of the smallest suitable bore catheter, refraining from daily meatal care with either povidone-iodine solution or soap and water because neither is proven to reduce the number of HUTI, and not changing catheters at arbitrary fixed intervals. The replacement of the collecting system when sterile closed drainage has been violated and separation of infected and uninfected patients with indwelling catheters may be useful, but this has not been proven in controlled trials.

Table 21.1 Methods to Avoid the Use of the Indwelling Catheter

Population	Methods
Postsurgical patients	Do not overhydrate
	Avoid anticholinergic drugs
	Provide urine containers at bedside
	Allow privacy and time to void
	Apply warm suprapubic pressure
	Consider drugs that stimulate the detrusor muscle and relax the sphincter
	Consider single catheterization if the patient does not void in 4 to 6 hours
Intensive care	Remove the indwelling catheter when stable
	Use intermittent catheterization as needed
	Condom catheters in males
Oliguric renal	Avoid catheterization; consider bedside ultrasound
Elderly, incontinent patients	Prompt voiding
	Absorbent perineal pads
	Condom catheters with penis prostheses, if needed
Neurogenic bladder	Intermittent catheterization
	Sphincterotomy and condom catheters, if needed
	Suprapubic catheters to void epididymitis

Continuous irrigation of the bladder with an antimicrobial solution or solution containing 0.25% acetic acid is no more effective than the closed drainage system and is not recommended. It is important to stress that prophylactic use of antibiotics sooner or later leads to the emergence of resistant strains and therefore should be avoided.

References

Kunin CM, McCormack RC. Prevention of catheter-induced urinary tract infections by sterile closed drainage. N Engl J Med 1966; 274:1155–61.

Wong ES. Guideline for prevention of catheter-associated urinary tract infections. Am J Med 1983;11:28–36.

Waren JW. Urinary tract infections. In: Wenzel RP, editor. Prevention and control of nosocomial infections. 3rd ed. Baltimore: Williams and Wilkins; 1997. p. 821–40.

CHAPTER 22

PNEUMONIA

Harald Seifert, MD

Key Issue: Nosocomial pneumonia is among the leading causes of hospital-acquired infections in both industrialized and developing countries and is associated with prolonged hospitalization and substantial morbidity and mortality. Accurate data regarding the epidemiology of nosocomial pneumonia is limited by the lack of a gold standard for diagnosis. Intubation and mechanical ventilation greatly increase the risk of nosocomial pneumonia. A considerable number of these infections can be prevented by simple infection control measures and proper disinfection of respiratory therapy equipment in patients requiring mechanical ventilation.

Known Facts

- *Streptococcus pneumoniae*, *Haemophilus influenzae*, and *Moraxella (Branhamella) catarrhalis* are the most common pathogens causing early onset nosocomial pneumonia (i.e., nosocomial pneumonia occurring during the first 3 days of hospital stay).
- Late-onset nosocomial pneumonia (i.e., nosocomial pneumonia occurring after the first 3 days of hospital stay) is usually polymicrobial in origin and mainly caused by *Staphylococcus aureus* and aerobic gram-negative bacilli such as *Pseudomonas aeruginosa*, *Enterobacter cloacae*, *Klebsiella pneumoniae*, *Serratia marcescens*, and *Acinetobacter baumannii*.
- Nosocomial pneumonia due to *Legionella pneumophila* may occur in hospitals with contaminated water supply.
- Diagnosis of nosocomial pneumonia is difficult and largely relies on clinical findings such as fever, cough, and development of purulent sputum, in combination with radiologic

evidence of a new or progressive pulmonary infiltrate, and cultures of sputum, tracheal aspirate, pleural fluid, and blood. Advanced diagnostic tools including bronchoscopic techniques, for example, quantitative culture of broncho-alveolar lavage, and protected specimen brush are mainly used in clinical research studies and are rarely available in developing countries.

- Nosocomial pneumonia is the leading cause of death due to nosocomial infections and has been associated with a crude mortality of ~30% and an attributable mortality of ~10% (one-third of the total mortality).

- Critically ill and intubated patients are at particular risk for nosocomial pneumonia.

- Cross-colonization plays a major role in the spread of noso-comial pathogens.

- Aspiration of bacteria from the oropharynx and the upper gastrointestinal tract into the tracheobronchial tree is the most common route of infection. Colonization of the stomach and the gastrointestinal tract is increased in patients with advanced age, achlorhydria, malnutrition, and use of antacids and H2-blockers that increase gastric pH. Tracheal colonization in the ventilated patient may result from leakage of bacteria around the cuff of the endotracheal tube. Bacteria can aggregate on the surface of the endotracheal tube over time and form a biofilm that protects the bacteria from the action of antimicrobial agents or host defenses.

- Host factors that predispose to nosocomial pneumonia include advanced age, severe acute or chronic underlying disease—in particular, chronic lung disease, prior surgery (thoracoabdominal procedures)—immunosuppression, depressed consciousness, obesity, malnutrition, and smoking.

- Factors increasing the risk for nosocomial pneumonia that enhance colonization of the oropharynx and that are largely preventable include bacterial cross infection from hospital personnel and colonized patients, improper disinfection of respiratory therapy equipment, resuscitation bags, spiro-meters, oxygen analyzers, and bronchoscopes, unrestrained use of antibiotics that may result in colonization with multi-drug-resistant organisms, medications that increase gastric pH, use of invasive devices, and use of sedatives.

Controversial Issues

- Selective decontamination of the digestive tract (SDD) with locally administered nonabsorbable antibiotic agents such as polymyxin, an aminoglycoside, or a quinolone coupled with an antifungal agent is a strategy to prevent bacterial coloniza-tion and lower respiratory tract infection of mechanically ventilated patients. Most clinical trials have demonstrated a decrease in the rates of nosocomial ventilator-associated pneumonia but had no effect on mortality. Furthermore, there are concerns regarding the development of antimicrobial resistance and superinfection with gram-positive bacteria.
- The value of systemic antimicrobial prophylaxis of nosoco-mial pneumonia has not been established, and the potential for superinfection with resistant organisms is a problem.
- Placement of a nasogastric tube may increase nasopharyn-geal colonization and cause reflux of gastric contents. It is unknown whether continuous or intermittent enteral feeding changes the risk of pneumonia.
- The maximum time that a ventilator circuit can be safely left unchanged on a patient has yet to be determined.

Suggested Practice

- Proper handwashing between patient contacts, and wearing gloves appropriately to prevent cross-contamination remains the most important infection control measure in mechanically ventilated patients.
- Thoroughly clean all equipment and devices to be sterilized or disinfected.
- Proper disinfection or sterilization of respiratory therapy equipment including resuscitation bags is important to pre-vent nosocomial pneumonia.

- Do not use cool-mist room air humidifiers without adequate sterilization or disinfection.
- Use only sterile fluids for nebulization and prevent contamination of medication nebulizers and humidifiers.
- Prevent backwash of contaminated tubing condensate into the tracheobronchial tree of mechanically ventilated patients.
- Do not routinely change ventilator circuits more often than every 48 hours.
- Assure proper suctioning practice and use sterile solutions to rinse the tracheal suction catheter.
- Prevent transfer of all kinds of equipment between patients.
- Maintain patient in a semirecumbent position, with head of bed elevated 30 degrees.
- Limit stress bleeding prophylaxis.
- Control pain that interferes with coughing and deep breathing in the immediate postoperative period by using systemic analgesia.
- Do not routinely use systemic antimicrobial agents to prevent nosocomial pneumonia.
- Consider isolating or cohorting patients with highly resistant organisms such as methicillin-resistant *Staphylococcus aureus* (MRSA).

References

Centers for Disease Control and Prevention. Guideline for prevention of nosocomial pneumonia. Infect Control Hosp Epidemiol 1994; 15:587–627.

Craven DE, Steger KA, Duncan RA. Prevention and control of nosocomial pneumonia. In: Wenzel RP, editor. Prevention and control of nosocomial infections. 3rd ed. Baltimore: Williams and Wilkins; 1997.

The American Thoracic Society. Hospital-acquired pneumonia in adults: diagnosis, assessment of severity, initial antimicrobial therapy, and preventive strategies. Am J Respir Crit Care Med 1995; 153:1711–25.

CHAPTER 23

DIPHTHERIA, TETANUS, PERTUSSIS

Richard P. Wenzel, MD, MSc

Key Issue: Diphtheria, tetanus, and pertussis can cause serious disease, and all are preventable with appropriate vaccination.

Known Facts

- *Corynebacterium diphtheriae*, a pleomorphic gram-positive rod, in the presence of a specific lysogenic beta phage, produces an endotoxin responsible for much of the disease. Person-to-person spread occurs by the respiratory route, although milkborne epidemics have been reported. Cutaneous diphtheria has been reported in alcoholics and in the homeless.

- *Bordetella pertussis* is a coccobacillary organism that causes whooping cough. Epidemic cycles occur every 3 to 5 years, and infection occurs in 50 to 100% of nonimmune individuals.

- *Clostridium tetani* is a gram-positive anaerobic rod that lives in the soil and produces a toxin that causes trismus (lockjaw) and violent muscle spasms.

Controversial Issues: There is no controversy about the value, efficacy, and cost benefit of routine immunization for diphtheria and tetanus. In some countries—but not in the United States—there is controversy about the frequency of the neurologic side effects of pertussis vaccines.

Suggested Practice: For children, three intramuscular doses of DPT vaccine should be administered at monthly intervals, beginning at 6 weeks of age. After age 7, the dT vaccine is recommended without the pertussis antigen. Boosters of dT should be given at 10-year intervals. For nonimmune persons and individuals exposed to tetanus, human tetanus immune globulin should be administered. It is also recommended as early therapy of tetanus.

All health care workers should have full immunization to diphtheria and tetanus and receive boosters with dT vaccine every 10 years.

Summary: Opportunities for routine immunization should be sought, such as during clinic visits by children and adults for any medical reason. In addition, there may be holidays or other celebrations which attract large numbers of people who might be available for immunization.

Isolation of those with diphtheria or pertussis should be attempted, and close contacts and family members should be sought for antibiotic prophylaxis and immunization, if necessary.

References

Fedson D. Immunization for healthcare workers and patients in hospitals. In: Wenzel RP, editor. Prevention and control of nosocomial infections. Baltimore: Williams & Wilkins; 1993. p. 214–94.

CHAPTER 24

MEASLES

Stephan Harbarth, MD, and Didier Pittet, MD, MS

Key Issue: Measles can cause serious disease and death. The disease is very readily communicable and can be prevented by appropriate immunization.

Known Facts:
- Since 1974 (the start of the World Health Organization [WHO]'s expanded immunization program), the number of cases and deaths attributed worldwide to measles has declined substantially, from an estimated 100 million cases and 5.8 million deaths in 1980 to an estimated 44 million cases and 1.1 million deaths in 1995. Despite recent achievements in measles immunization coverage, measles remains one of the leading causes of child mortality in developing countries, responsible for approximately 10% of all deaths among malnourished children aged less than 5 years.
- The prevention of measles is important because the disease may result in such complications as middle ear infections, laryngotracheitis, pneumonia, gastroenteritis, and encephalitis. Survivors of encephalitis often suffer permanent brain damage and mental retardation. Encephalitis and death from respiratory and neurologic causes ensue in approximately 1 of 1000 reported cases of measles. The risk of severe complications and death is greater among infants and adults than among children and adolescents.
- The consequences of transmission of measles in a hospital include not only the related morbidity and mortality but also the significant cost of evaluating and containing an outbreak and the marked disruption of regular hospital routine.

Controversial Issues

- There is ongoing controversy about the frequency and importance of the side effects of the measles vaccine, such as aseptic meningitis, Guillain-Barré syndrome, and inflammatory bowel disease.
- A recently published article by Shaheen et al. suggested that measles may prevent the development of atopy in African children surviving the infection.
- A community study from Senegal did not observe any long-term mortality after measles infection and documented a lower mortality in infected patients than in uninfected, unvaccinated children.

Suggested Practice

- No specific treatment for measles is available but active immunization with live vaccine confers immunity which is probably lifelong. In developed countries, it is usually given as part of the MMR (measles-mumps-rubella) vaccine at 15 to 18 months of age and one dose again in childhood. In developing countries, in which the incidence of natural measles before the age of 1 year is high, live vaccines may be given at 6 to 9 months of age but should be followed by additional routine doses.
- Passive immunization with immune globulin is recommended for those who are susceptible to measles and who are at high risk of severe or fatal infection (children with cell-mediated immunity defects or malignancy). The immune globulin should be given within 6 days of exposure to measles.
- In the hospital setting, screening for measles immunity followed by direct immunization is less expensive than immunizing all potentially susceptible employees.

Summary: Because of the ease of transmission of measles, and because measles may cause severe disease in children and adults, routine immunization should be given to children.

Measles vaccine induces seroconversion in over 90% of susceptible persons with a single dose. Hospital patients with suspected or confirmed measles should be placed in isolation as a precaution to prevent droplet transmission until 4 days after the onset of rash.

References

Aaby P, Samb B, Andersen M, Simondon F. No long-term excess mortality after measles infection: a community study from Senegal. Am J Epidemiol 1996;143:1035–41.

CDC/MMWR; Recommendations and Reports. Measles eradication: Recommendations from a meeting cosponsored by the WHO, the PAHO, and CDC. 1997, Vol 46, RR-11.

Krause PJ, Gross PA, Barrett TL, Dellinger EP, Martone WJ, McGowan JE, et al. Quality standard for assurance of measles immunity among health care workers. Infect Control Hosp Epidemiol 1994; 15:193–9.

Williams WW, Atkinson WA, Holmes SJ, Orenstein WA. Nosocomial measles, mumps, rubella and other viral infections. In: Mayhall CG, editor. Hospital Epidemiology and Infection Control. Baltimore: William and Wilkins; 1996. p. 523–35.

World Health Organization. Expanded programme on immunization—accelerated measles strategies. Wkly Epidemiol Rec 1994;69: 229–34.

CHAPTER 25

Blood Transfusions and Intravenous Fluids

Timothy F. Brewer, MD, MPH

Key Issues: Blood transfusions and intravenous fluid replacement, when indicated, may be life-saving procedures. However, many developing countries and least developed countries do not have the resources to appropriately screen blood for infectious agents, match blood groups between donors and recipients, and store blood and blood components for future use. These countries also often lack adequate supplies of sterile needles, tubing, and other equipment necessary to safely administer blood products or intravenous fluids. In these settings, blood transfusions and, to a much lesser extent, intravenous fluids may be an important cause of transmission of infectious diseases to patients.

Known Facts

- Using repeat, volunteer blood donors, instead of paid donors or replacement donors, lowers the risk of infections in the blood transfusions.
- Donor deferral has been shown to reduce the rate of human immunodeficiency virus (HIV) and hepatitis in transfused blood.
- When properly done, blood group matching and screening with supplemental testing for HIV, hepatitis B and C viruses (HBV, HCV), and other pathogens reduces the mortality risk from a blood transfusion to under 1 in 100,000 patients.
- Skin flora (coagulase-negative staphylococci, diphtheroids, or *Staphylococcus aureus*) entering the catheter insertion site and colonizing the catheter are the most common infection associated with intravenous fluid use.
- The risk of infection increases with the length of time the catheter is left in place.

- Contaminated intravenous fluids, often by gram-negative bacilli, are associated with high rates of bacteremia in patients.

Controversial Issue
- Whether screening for hepatitis B surface antigen is cost effective in endemic populations is undetermined.

Suggested Practice

Intravenous (IV) Fluids.
- Always wash hands thoroughly (15 to 20 seconds) before inserting IV catheters, preparing infusion fluids including adding medications, or changing dressings.
- Disinfect the skin with 10% alcoholic povidone-iodine or 70% isopropyl alcohol before catheter insertion. The skin should not be touched once it has been prepared ("no-touch" technique). Choose a site on an upper extremity which will minimize patient discomfort and restriction of movement. Avoid the groin, lower extremities, and bony prominences because these sites have higher rates of infection and/or discomfort. Wear nonsterile gloves when inserting peripheral lines.
- Medication ports should be disinfected with 70% isopropyl alcohol before medicines are added to IV fluids using the no-touch technique.
- Sterile needles and tubing must be used for all IV fluid administrations. Whenever possible, disposable needles and tubing should be used. Inspect IV fluid containers for cracks, leaks, or cloudiness. Give only sterile fluid and medicines intravenously. Medicines should be added to IV fluids only by trained personnel, preferably in the pharmacy under aseptic conditions.
- Secure the catheter to prevent movement, and cover the insertion site with a sterile dressing. Check the site daily. Change dressing only when necessary. If possible, remove or rotate peripheral IV catheters to a new site every 72 hours.

Blood Transfusions.

- Use the same general techniques as recommended for IV fluids.
- Use IV fluids instead of blood for volume resuscitation, whenever possible.
- Screen donors and blood to reduce the risk of transmitting infectious diseases (Tables 25.1 and 25.2).
- All blood products should be assumed to be infectious and should be handled with gloves.
- No medications should be added to blood transfusions. Tubing used for transfusions should not be reused because of the risk of inadequate sterilization.
- Monitor the patient's temperature and blood pressure during transfusion. Stop the transfusion immediately if fever or hypotension occurs as these may be signs of a noninfectious immune reaction.

Summary: Hemorrhage during delivery or secondary to trauma, and acute hemolytic anemia from malaria or sickle cell crisis are common indications for transfusions in developing countries. With the advent of modern blood banking technology and the introduction of screening tests for infectious diseases, blood transfusions in most developed market economy countries are very safe. The most commonly transfused infectious agent in developed countries is hepatitis C virus (HCV). With the use of second- and third-generation enzyme immunoassays for HCV, however, the risk of post-transfusion HCV has dropped to less than 1%. In contrast, the risk of human immunodeficiency virus 1 (HIV-1) may be as low as 1 in 450,000 to 600,000 units in countries such as the United States.

In developing countries, blood transfusions remain a significant source of HIV-1 transmission. According to a World Health Organization survey, in 1992, less than half (46%) the least developed countries screened all blood donations for HIV-1. Other pathogens transmitted by blood transfusions include HCV, HBV, human T-cell lymphotrophic virus types I and II (HTLV-I and II), cytomegalovirus, Epstein-Barr virus, delta hepatitis, malaria, babesiosis, toxoplasmosis, leishmaniasis, syphilis, and a variety of bacterial contaminants. Though screening tests exist for many of these pathogens, the tests are

---

Table 25.1 Donor Deferral for Low-Resource Countries with Limited or No Blood Screening

All

Donors should be in good general health without signs or symptoms of infectious diseases including fever, jaundice, diarrhea, lymphadenopathy, hepatosplenomegaly, or genital ulcers

Limited Blood Supply (reliance on replacement donors and no blood storage facilities)

Persons with known HIV, Chagas' disease, chronic hepatitis (HBV carriers), visceral leishmaniasis, or untreated malaria
Persons with stigmata or history of intravenous drug use

Moderate Blood Supply (donor pool and/or some blood storage facilities)

Recent sexual contacts of persons with HIV or hepatitis
Persons with a history of sexually transmitted diseases or hepatitis

Reasonable Blood Supply (volunteer donor pool and blood storage facilities)

Follow the American Association of Blood Banks Criteria for Protecting Donor Recipients
  Permanent Deferral
    Alcoholism or stigmata of intravenous drug use
    Hepatitis after age 11
    High-risk group for HIV-1/2
    History of babesiosis or Chagas' disease
    Recipients of human pituitary growth hormone
    Positive for HIV-1/2, HBsAg, anti-HBc antibody, anti-HCV, or anti-HTLV I/II
  1-year Deferral
    Recipients of potentially infected blood or tissue products
    Recipients of rabies vaccine after at-risk animal bite
    Treatment for syphilis or gonorrhea
    Sexual contact with persons with HIV, hepatitis, or at high risk for HIV
    Application of a tattoo, ear or body piercing, or acupuncture
    Contaminated needlestick injuries or mucous membrane exposure to blood

Adapted from Schleupner CJ. Protecting recipients of blood and blood products. In: Wenzel RP, editor. Prevention and control of nosocomial infections. 3rd ed. Baltimore: Williams and Wilkins; 1997. p. 1187–214.
HBsAg = hepatitis B surface antigen; HBc = hepatitis B core

relatively expensive and require trained staff and equipment not found in many hospitals and clinics. These health care institutions also often do not have the staff or equipment to do blood group matching, separation of whole blood into components, or long-term storage. Because of inadequate blood supplies, some hospitals and clinics rely on replacement donations. In this situation, family members donate blood to replace units used for the patient. Replacement donations are more likely to transmit infections than those obtained from voluntary, repeat donors.

Despite the risk of both noninfectious and infectious complications from blood transfusions in developing countries, in certain circumstances transfusions are a life-saving intervention. Donor screening should decrease the risk of transfusing infected units of blood in these circumstances (Table 25.1). Long-term solutions include the development of volunteer, low-risk blood donor pools to improve the supply of lower-risk blood and simpler low-cost blood banking technologies and screening tests for use in developing countries.

Intravenous fluids are much less likely to transmit infections than blood transfusions, and should be used instead of transfusions when emergency volume expansion is needed.

Table 25.2 Screening Tests for Infectious Diseases Transmitted by Blood and Blood Products

Serologic Test (in likely decreasing order of importance)*
HIV-1 antibody (EIA)
HBsAg (RIA or EIA)
Anti-HCV (EIA)
HIV-1/2 antibody (EIA)
HTLV-I/II antibody (EIA)
Nontreponemal test (RPR, etc.)
HIV-1 p24 antigen (EIA)

*The exact order depends on the prevalence of the relative diseases in the community and the efficacy of donor deferral.

EIA = enzyme immunoassay; RIA = radioimmunoassay ; RPR = rapid plasma reagin

Severe dehydration in patients unable to take oral rehydration and volume loss due to hemorrhage are situations when IV fluids could be used. Catheter-related infections are the most common infectious complication of IV therapy. Gram-negative sepsis from infusing contaminated fluids, though uncommon, can be a fatal complication. It is essential that only sterile IV fluids and tubing be used.

References

Gibbs WN, Corcoran P. Blood safety in developing countries. Vox Sang 1994;67:377–81.

Prince AM. Control of hepatitis B virus infection in third-world countries. Transfus Med Rev 1990;4:187–90.

Schleupner CS. Protecting recipients of blood and blood products. In: Wenzel RP, editor. Prevention and control of nosocomial infections. 3rd ed. Baltimore: Williams and Wilkins; 1997. p. 1187–214.

CHAPTER 26

MECHANICAL VENTILATION

Stephan Harbarth, MD, and Didier Pittet, MD, MS

Key Issue: Mechanical ventilation is the main risk factor for nosocomial pneumonia in critically ill patients.

Known Facts: Ventilator-associated pneumonia is the most common nosocomial infection (NI) in intensive care units (ICUs), accounting for approximately 30 to 50% of all ICU-acquired infections. Ventilator-associated pneumonia is associated with a high crude mortality rate and an attributable mortality around 10% in critically ill patients. In surviving patients, it causes substantial morbidity, prolongs the length of stay in the hospital, and therefore considerably increases resource utilization.

Controversial Issues

- Diagnosis of ventilator-associated pneumonia is one of the most controversial issues. Fever, leukocytosis, and lung consolidation, hallmarks of pneumonia in otherwise healthy patients, can result from other pathogenic mechanisms in intubated patients, such as pulmonary edema, contusion, atelectasis, pleural effusions, and acute respiratory distress syndrome (ARDS).

- Invasive techniques to diagnose ventilator-associated pneumonia include protected bronchoalveolar lavage (BAL), nonbronchoscopic ("blind") BAL, and "blind" protected specimen brush. The use of any of these techniques should be strongly encouraged to increase the accuracy of the difficult diagnosis of ventilator-associated pneumonia.

- Selective digestive decontamination (SDD) has been studied for many years and involves the use of topical oral and intestinal antibiotics, often with a systemic antibiotic added for the first few days of the regimen, with the goal being the elimination of all potential pathogens from the gastrointestinal tract. With sterilization of endogenous bacterial sources, infection may be avoided. In spite of the data from many clinical trials, it is difficult to recommend confidently whether or not SDD should be routinely used in the ICU setting. However, it may be premature to ignore the potential benefits of SDD because the results of most clinical trials of SDD were encouraging in reducing infection rates.

- Other unresolved issues for the prevention of ventilator-associated pneumonia include placing filters in the breathing circuit to collect condensate or bacterial filters in the breathing system; frequency of changing devices while being used on one patient; and wearing sterile gloves rather than unsterile gloves when suctioning secretions.

Suggested Practice: A number of preventive strategies have been applied and are strongly recommended for all hospitals:

- Education and training of health care workers.
- Surveillance of high-risk patients to determine trends and outbreaks of ventilator-associated pneumonia within the ICU.
- Different measures to interrupt exogenous transmission of microorganisms (disinfection and appropriate maintenance of equipment, use of sterile water for rinsing reusable equipment, change of breathing circuits not more than once within 48 hours, periodical drainage of condensate in the tubing of a breathing circuit, barrier precautions for handling respiratory secretions, and handwashing).
- The use of appropriate techniques to diagnose ventilator-associated pneumonia should be encouraged to reduce overuse of antimicrobial agents which can increase antibiotic resistance.
- Bacterial colonization of the oropharynx with aerobic gram-negative bacilli and microaspiration of these colonized oropharyngeal contents to the lower airways are probably

the most important circumstances leading to the development of ventilator-associated pneumonia. A variety of strategies are recommended to prevent aspiration associated with enteral feeding: elevation of the head at an angle of 30 to 45 degrees, discontinuation of enteral tube feeding and removal of devices as soon as possible, routine verification of the placement of the feeding tube and the patient's intestinal motility, and the installation of an effective drainage of subglottic secretions.

• To prevent gastric and oropharyngeal colonization, several prospective studies demonstrated lower rates of ventilator-associated pneumonia in patients randomized to receive sucralfate for stress ulcer prophylaxis compared with those patients receiving antacids or histamine-2-receptor antagonists.

Summary: Traditional preventive measures for ventilator-associated pneumonia include decreasing the risk of aspiration by the patient, preventing cross-contamination or colonization via hands of personnel, appropriate disinfection or sterilization of respiratory devices, and education of hospital staff. New measures being investigated involve reducing oropharyngeal and gastric colonization by pathogenic microorganisms. However, the benefit of this strategy remains controversial and may facilitate the emergence of resistant microorganisms. In contrast, non-pharmacologic methods designed to reduce gastroesophageal reflux, tracheal aspiration, and direct inoculation of microorganisms into the lower respiratory tract can be applied in a routine way in mechanically ventilated patients and are effective in reducing the incidence of ventilator-associated pneumonia. Effective drainage of subglottic secretions, elevation of the head of the bed, and careful handling of the artificial airway such as periodic monitoring of the intracuff pressure are inexpensive and effective measures to prevent ventilator-associated pneumonia.

References

Guidelines for Prevention of Nosocomial Pneumonia. CDC/MMWR recommendations and reports, 1997. Vol 46, RR-1.

Hospital-acquired pneumonia in adults: diagnosis, assessment of severity, initial antimicrobial therapy, and preventive strategies. A consensus statement by the American Thoracic Society. Am J Respir Crit Care Med 1995;153:1711–25.

Pittet D, Harbarth S. The intensive care unit. In: Bennett J, Brachman P, editors. Nosocomial Infections. 4th ed. 1998. p. 381–402.

CHAPTER 27

PREPARING THE PATIENT FOR SURGERY

Helen Giamarellou, MD

Key Issue: Appropriate skin preparation plus antimicrobial prophylaxis can decrease the incidence of both superficial and deep wound infections after certain operations.

Known Facts: A preoperative shower, preparation of the skin with antiseptics in the operating room, and a single preoperative dose of a first- or second-generation cephalosporin are extremely important to significantly decrease wound infection rates. Regrettably, several postoperative doses of prophylaxis are generally administered in some medical centers leading to excess cost and the emergence of multiresistant bacteria.

Controversial Issues

- Hair removal from the operative site is still disputed. The duration of prophylaxis in the trauma patient is not well defined. Assessment of risk factors in clean operations requires more studies.

Suggested Practice: The goal of antimicrobial prophylaxis in surgery is to prevent both superficial and deep surgical site infections. Surgical antimicrobial prophylaxis has been shown in many randomized clinical trials to reduce significantly the incidence of postoperative wound infections. The following principles of prophylaxis should be applied:

- A single, full therapeutic dose of antibiotic should be given intravenously immediately before skin incision and simultaneously with the induction of anesthesia, i.e., prior to tissue contamination to ensure effective tissue concentrations throughout the operative period. Antibiotics are most effective when given before inoculation of bacteria. They are ineffective if given three to four hours after inoculation.

- In most clean and clean-contaminated cases, including those involving the surgical placement of foreign material, cefazolin alone should be administered upon induction of anesthesia and skin incision. In contaminated operations, cefazolin plus an agent active against anaerobes should be used.

- The selection of the appropriate drug should be based on the most likely bacteria to cause infection in each situation. A single drug should be used, whenever possible. Cephalosporins, in particular, cefazolin, is ideal for prophylaxis because of its broad spectrum of activity, the moderately long serum half-life, low toxicity, ease of administration, and low cost. Third-generation cephalosporins are more costly and promote the emergence of resistant strains. In general, they should not be used for routine prophylaxis. Since coverage against both aerobic and anaerobic gram-negative organisms is necessary for colorectal surgery, penetrating abdominal trauma, or primary appendectomy, cefoxitin or cefotetan are recommended as single agents. For patients with beta-lactam allergies, metronidazole and gentamicin can be used.

- Prophylaxis should not be extended beyond 24 hours following surgery. As long as adequate serum drug levels are maintained during the operation, a single dose is as effective as multiple doses.

- In the case of massive hemorrhage, or whenever the duration of an operation exceeds 3 hours, a repeat dose should be given every two to three half-lives.

- Prophylactic antibiotics are indicated in cases of placement of prosthetic materials (e.g., heart valves, vascular grafts, orthopedic hardware) or whenever host-risk factors suggest the need for prophylaxis. Since staphylococci are the major threat in infected prostheses, vancomycin should be used in institutions with a high predominance of methicillin-resistant strains.

Summary: Preparation of patients for surgery aimed at preventing postoperative wound infection is based on appropriate skin preparation and antimicrobial prophylaxis.

Decontamination of the skin preoperatively is very important to prevent wound infection, particularly in clean procedures. A preoperative shower with an antiseptic soap seems to reduce the incidence of postoperative infections. Chlorhexidine gluconate was significantly superior when compared to povidone-iodine and triclocarban medicated soap showers. Hair removal at the operative site by shaving, particularly the night before surgery, should be abandoned since shaving produces significant injury. Subsequently, the injured skin sites are colonized and serve as a niche of bacterial contamination of surgical wounds. The risk of wound infections from clippers or a depilatory have been found to be lower than that from shaving. Interestingly, patients with no hair removal may have even lower rates of wound infection. Skin preparation in the operating room should be performed by trained personnel. The prep starts with a careful cleansing of the operative site with a detergent (with or without a degreasing agent). The antiseptic is applied in concentric circles starting at the proposed operative incision site. Chlorhexidine gluconate or an iodophor scrub are usually used.

Wound infection has been defined as purulent discharge from an incision, regardless of whether organisms are cultured. In 1992, the CDC redefined the term as "surgical site infections," and divided them into superficial and deep infections. The superficial infections involve only the skin and subcutaneous tissues while deep infections involve at least muscle and fascial layers. Incisions may be contaminated by the patient's own normal flora or by flora from the environment, including the operative team. Correct surveillance of wound infection extends to 30 days following surgery. In the case of implants, surveillance is extended for up to 1 year.

The traditional surgical wound classification system was established based on the exposure of the incision to bacterial contamination (Table 27.1). Infection was reported in 3.3% of clean wounds, in 10.8% of clean-contaminated, in 16.3% of contaminated, and in 28.6% of dirty wounds. In the Study of the Efficacy of Nosocomial Infection Control (SENIC), a new classification based on patients' risk assessment rather than wounds was developed. Risk factors included abdominal operations, operations exceeding 2 hours, and having three or more associated discharge diagnoses. Patients with no risk factors were at low risk for infection (1%), those with one factor at moderate risk (3.6%), and those with two or more factors at

---

Table 27.1 Classification of Surgical Wounds

Clean

No entry into the gastrointestinal, respiratory, or genitourinary tracts

No signs of acute inflammation or infection

Nontraumatic

No violations of aseptic technique

Clean-Contaminated

Entry into the gastrointestinal or respiratory tract without significant contamination

Biliary tract entered in the absence of infected bile

Oropharynx or vagina entered

Genitourinary tract entered in the absence of infected urine

Minor violation of aseptic technique

Contaminated

Major contamination following entry into the gastroinestinal or respiratory tracts

Entrance of genitourinary or biliary tracts in the presence of acute infection

Fresh traumatic wounds

Major break in aseptic technique

Dirty

Acute bacterial inflammation or pus encountered

Perforated viscus encountered

Traumatic wound with retained devitalized tissue, foreign material, fecal contamination, and/or delayed treatment

high risk (8.9 to 27%). The National Nosocomial Infection Surveillance (NNIS) system, in 1991, attempted to redefine risk factors. The following risk factors provided a greater discrimination for the patient at risk of wound infection: (1) a contaminated or dirty wound class; (2) high preoperative risk as defined by an American Society of Anesthesiologists (ASA) preoperative assessment score of three or more; and (3) a duration of operation exceeding the 75th percentile for a given procedure. Long operations generally include greater blood loss, increased complexity, and violations of asepsis. Malnutrition, advanced age, obesity, diabetes mellitus, malignancy, and the use of steroids or immunosuppressive drugs are also risk factors for wound infection.

Appropriate antibiotic prophylaxis reduces morbidity and costs by preventing surgical site infections. However, it should be emphasized that antibiotic overuse and misuse for surgical prophylaxis accounts for as many as half of all antibiotics costs prescribed in US hospitals, and contributes to the emergence of multidrug-resistant microorganisms.

References

Antimicrobial prophylaxis in surgery. Med Lett Drugs Ther 1993; 35:91–4.

Classen DC, Evans RS, Restomik SL, et al. The timing of prophylactic administration of antibiotics and the risk of surgical wound infection. N Engl J Med 1992;326:281–6.

Malangoni MA, editor. Critical issues in operating room management. Philadelphia; Lippincott-Raven; 1997.

CHAPTER 28

INFECTION CONTROL IN OBSTETRICS

J. A. J. W. Kluytmans, MD, PhD

Key Issue: Neonatal sepsis and postpartum endometritis can be largely prevented by simple infection control measures. However, in developing countries, they still cause substantial morbidity and mortality. Most infections are caused by microorganisms of the mothers' vaginal flora.

Known Facts

- The most important microorganisms causing neonatal sepsis are group B streptococci (GBS) and *E. coli*.
- Cleansing of the birth canal with an antiseptic reduces the neonatal infection rate.
- Prevention of infections with GBS can be achieved by screening and treating vaginal colonization during pregnancy. The cost-effectiveness of this strategy depends on the setting.
- Cesarean section is associated with a higher rate of postpartum endometritis (10 to 20%) than vaginal delivery.
- Cleansing of the birth canal with a disinfectant during vaginal examinations reduces the risk of postpartum endometritis.
- Single-dose antibiotic prophylaxis reduces the risk for postpartum endometritis after cesarean section in high-risk patients.
- Although rare, outbreaks of classical childbed fever caused by group A hemolytic streptococci do occur and warrant prompt investigations into the source. This includes searching for carriers.
- During labor there may be frequent and uncontrolled contact with blood and other body fluids. Preventive measures are necessary to avoid transmission of bloodborne pathogens.

Controversial Issues

- The value of antibiotic prophylaxis in women undergoing cesarean section who are not in labor and have intact membranes is unclear.
- Compared with cesarean section, symphysiolysis is supposed to be associated with a lower rate of postpartum endometritis.

Suggested Practice

- General infection control measures should be taken before, during, and after labor.
- During labor, gloves should be worn at all times. It is advisable to wear a gown, mask, and eye protection.
- During vaginal examinations, the birth canal should be cleansed with a disinfectant.
- In high-risk patients, single-dose antibiotic prophylaxis should be administered when cesarean section is performed. Antibiotics should be given directly after the umbilical cord has been clamped.

Summary: The importance of infection control in obstetrics was established when Semmelweis made his historic observations during the second half of the nineteenth century. Nowadays, in developed countries, most infectious complications of delivery are prevented. However, in developing countries, neonatal and maternal postpartum morbidity and mortality due to bacterial infections are substantial. In areas with a high prevalence of human immunodeficiency virus (HIV) infection, the morbidity and mortality rates have further increased. Simple infection control measures can prevent infectious complications to a large extent. For instance, cleansing of the birth canal with 0.25% chlorhexidine at every vaginal examination before delivery, combined with a wipe of the newborn, results in a significant decrease of neonatal and maternal infections and neonatal mortality, at a cost of less than US $0.10 per patient.

Neonatal sepsis. The most important pathogens causing neonatal sepsis are group B streptococci (GBS) and *Escherichia coli*. The newborn is considered to be colonized during passage through the birth canal. Although disputable, newborn infections which are thus acquired are considered nosocomial. Cleansing of the birth canal with an antiseptic, as mentioned earlier, results in a decrease of neonatal infections. Prevention of infections with GBS can be achieved by screening and treating vaginal colonization during pregnancy.

Two prevention strategies for the prevention of neonatal GBS sepsis consist of giving intrapartum antibiotic prophylaxis to women

1. who are identified as GBS carriers through screening cultures collected at 35 to 37 weeks' gestation or to women who develop premature labor or rupture of the membranes before 37 weeks gestation; and
2. who develop one or more of the following risk factors at the time of labor: delivery at <37 weeks' gestation, membrane rupture for >18 hours, or intrapartum temperature >100.4°F.

Prophylaxis should be considered for women who had children with GBS sepsis after previous childbirths and women who had GBS bacteriuria earlier in the course of pregnancy.

Postpartum Endometritis. Postpartum endometritis is a serious complication of delivery. Most infections are caused by microorganisms which are part of the mother's endogenous flora. Outbreaks are rare. Prevention depends largely on the elimination of risk factors. Cesarean section is associated with a higher rate of postpartum endometritis than vaginal delivery. In developing countries, there is an ongoing discussion whether symphysiolysis should be preferred over cesarean section when the latter is associated with a high postpartum endometritis rate.

Well-documented risk factors for postpartum endometritis after cesarean section include membrane rupture, labor, low socioeconomic status, and frequent vaginal examinations.

Well-documented risk factors for postpartum endometritis after vaginal delivery include prolonged membrane rupture, midforceps delivery, anemia, maternal soft tissue trauma, and bacterial vaginosis. Cleansing of the birth canal with a disinfectant during vaginal examinations reduces the risk of postpartum endometritis. Single-dose antibiotic prophylaxis after clamping the umbilical cord reduces the risk for postpartum endometritis after cesarean section in high-risk patients.

Bloodborne pathogens are a threat to mother, child, and health care worker during delivery. Scalp electrodes are contraindicated if the mother is infected with hepatitis B or C, or HIV. In mothers with hepatitis B the newborn should be immunized after delivery, and in mothers infected with HIV, antiretroviral therapy during pregnancy reduces the risk of transmission to the newborn. Blood exposure occurs frequently during labor. Gloves should be worn at all times, and it is advisable to wear gowns, masks, and eye protection.

Herpes Simplex Virus (HSV). Mothers with active genital HSV infections should be handled with barrier precautions. Health care workers and the mother should wear gloves when touching the infected area or materials (gauzes etc.).

References

Mead PB, Hess SM, Page SD. Prevention and control of nosocomial infections in obstetrics and gynecology. In: Wenzel RP, editor. Prevention and control of nosocomial infections. 3rd ed. Philadelphia: Williams and Wilkins; 1997. p. 995–1016.

Taha TE, Biggar RJ, Broadhead RL, et al. Effect of cleansing the birth canal with antiseptic solution on maternal and newborn morbidity and mortality in Malawi: clinical trial. BMJ 1997;315:216–20.

CHAPTER 29

STREPTOCOCCUS PYOGENES

Alice H. M. Wong, MD, and Michael T. Wong, NM, MD

Key Issues: Handwashing is one of the most important infection control practices for the prevention of spread of infection with *Streptococcus pyogenes* (*S. pyogenes*).

Known Facts

- The most common site of carriage is the pharynx. Other possible sites include the skin, rectum, and vagina.
- Transmission occurs primarily via direct contact with patients or carriers and via large respiratory droplets. Fomites as a source of transmission are common.
- A variety of clinical presentations of *S. pyogenes* infection may occur including pharyngitis, otitis media, quinsy, skin and soft tissue infections (pyoderma, impetigo, erysipelas, and scarlet fever), pneumonia, and puerperal fever. More recently, invasive infection such as necrotizing fasciitis associated with the streptococcal toxic shock syndrome has acquired prominence.
- Postinfectious complications include acute rheumatic fever with secondary mitral or aortic valve injury and acute glomerulonephritis (GN). It is important to note that while infection with pharyngeal strains may result in either syndrome, infection with skin strains are only associated with acute GN.
- *S. pyogenes* is an infrequent cause of outbreaks of nosocomial infection but may result in explosive outbreaks of pharyngitis or impetigo in school-aged children or in group settings.
- Streptococcal infections should be treated to limit the development of secondary complications.
- Eradication of the carrier state may be difficult.

Controversial Issues

- The frequency and duration of follow-up cultures after an attempt to eradicate *S. pyogenes* colonization is unclear.

Suggested Practice

- Wear gloves and gowns for contact with the patient's skin lesions, wounds, and purulent discharge. Discard the gloves after use and wash hands thoroughly between patient contacts. Contact isolation may be discontinued after 24 hours of directed antistreptococcal therapy.
- Health care workers who are known or suspected to have infection or colonization of their respiratory tract with *S. pyogenes* should wear a mask to reduce respiratory spread of their organisms.
- Attempt to eradicate colonization in those health care workers who are proven sources of outbreaks.
- Control of a persistent outbreak may require the prophylaxis of all uninfected patients with penicillin V K.

Summary: *Streptococcus pyogenes* (group A β-hemolytic streptococcus) is a gram-positive, chaining, catalase-negative coccus. The pharynx, skin, rectum, and vagina are all possible sites of carriage. Infection with *S. pyogenes* has a variety of clinical presentations. The most severe of these is the critically ill patient with streptococcal toxic shock syndrome or with puerperal fever with sepsis. In health care institutions, nosocomial outbreaks of postoperative wound, burn wound, and puerperal infections have all been documented. Bacteremia related to intravascular catheter insertion and pneumonia have also been described.

Direct contact with patients or carriers and large respiratory droplets are the primary means of acquisition. Disease caused by *S. pyogenes* is the most common in late winter and early spring. Explosive outbreaks may occur in the community during these months, while skin infections are common year-round in the tropics. Although respiratory tract carriage of this organism is common, the respiratory route is not the only source of transmission.

When more than one case of nosocomially acquired *S. pyogenes* is documented, an outbreak investigation should be initiated. With the development of case definitions, active case finding should take place. The organisms isolated should be typed to ascertain whether or not they are from a common source. The most commonly described sources of surgical site infection have been rectal or vaginal carriage. Health care workers or patients identified as being possible sources of the outbreak should have pharyngeal, rectal, and vaginal cultures performed. In addition, they should be examined for evidence of dermatitis. Symptomatic individuals should be treated promptly.

Contaminated hands of health care workers are another important means of transmission, particularly outside of the setting of the operating room. Appropriate gloving and good handwashing techniques are important to emphasize in efforts to control an outbreak. Occasionally, control of a persistent outbreak may require the prophylaxis of all uninfected patients with penicillin. With the identification of a source for the outbreak, an attempt should be made to decolonize the individual. Penicillin is not effective in this instance. Erythromycin, clindamycin, or rifampin may be used once the susceptibility pattern of the isolate becomes available. It is important to note that erythromycin resistance is a problem in some locations. Follow-up cultures should be performed as some individuals become recolonized after an attempt at eradication. It is unclear as to how long these individuals need to be followed up.

Prompt identification and investigation of an outbreak of nosocomial *S. pyogenes* infection will assist in its control. Rapid diagnosis and treatment of *S. pyogenes* infections will reduce the frequency of postinfectious complications. The importance of good handwashing practices cannot be overemphasized.

References

Streptococcal diseases caused by group A (beta hemolytic) streptococci. In: Benenson AS, editor. Control of communicable disease manual. 16th ed. Baltimore: United Book Press; 1995. p. 438–45.

Bisno AL, Stevens DL. Streptococcal infections of skin and soft tissues. N Engl J Med 1996;334:240–5.

Crossley K. Streptococci. In: Mayhall CG, editor. Hospital epidemiology and infection control. Baltimore: Williams and Wilkins; 1996: 326–34.

CHAPTER 30

Staphylococcus Aureus

Werner E. Bischoff, MD, and Michael B. Edmond, MD, MPH

Key Issue: *Staphylococcus aureus* is a major human pathogen that commonly causes nosocomial and community-acquired infections. It is a highly virulent organism and is exhibiting increasing antibiotic resistance.

Known Facts

- Up to 30% of healthy people carry *S. aureus* in their anterior nares and other hairy or moist body areas.
- *S. aureus* causes approximately 12% of all hospital-acquired infections in the United States.
- The most common sites of nosocomial *S. aureus* infections are respiratory tract (20%) and surgical wounds (19%), followed by other sites such as bloodstream and urinary tract.
- Regarding antimicrobial resistance patterns, *S. aureus* can be divided into methicillin-susceptible *S. aureus* (MSSA) and methicillin-resistant *S. aureus* (MRSA).
- MSSA strains are mostly acquired in the community whereas MRSA has its major source and reservoir in health care facilities.
- Risk factors for MSSA/MRSA colonization and infection include underlying diseases (respiratory infections, diabetes mellitus, dialysis, allergy therapy, conditions causing loss of skin integrity such as eczema or burns), prolonged hospitalization, IV drug use, prior antimicrobial therapy, and exposure to other infected or colonized individuals.
- Major route of transmission is contact; airborne transmission is uncommon.

Controversial Issues

- The rate of hospital-acquired MSSA infections might be underestimated due to focusing on MRSA.

- No proven efficacy of intervention methods such as MRSA screening on admission or routine surveillance cultures and decolonization of patients or staff.

Suggested Practice

MSSA

- Administer routine perioperative antibiotic prophylaxis.
- Use standard precautions.

MRSA

- Use barrier (contact) precautions.
- Enforce handwashing with antiseptic agents, e.g., chlorhexidine gluconate or alcohol for staff, visitors, and infected or colonized patients.
- Provide private room or cohorting with other MRSA patients
- Offer decolonization with intranasal mupirocin for patients with recurring infections and for colonized personnel.
- Maintain a reference list of MRSA patients in case of re-admission.
- If MRSA patient is transferred, notify receiving health care facility.
- No special precautions for home discharge are required—emphasize good handwashing.

Summary: In the community, *S. aureus* is best known as the cause of furuncles and soft tissue infections. In the hospital environment, *S. aureus* may cause life-threatening infections such as pneumonia or surgical site infections. With the emergence of methicillin resistance in Europe and subsequent worldwide spread, *S. aureus* has become one of the most important nosocomial pathogens.

Methicillin-susceptible *S. aureus* and methicillin-resistant *S. aureus* have equivalent potential for colonization and infection. The risk factors for acquisition of *S. aureus* are influenced by age, general health status, and external factors such as prolonged hospitalization or exposure to colonized or infected individuals. The nares are the usual reservoir for *S. aureus* but other locations such as moist or hairy body areas, skin defects, wounds, and burns also can be colonized. Methicillin-resistant *S. aureus* carriage may be eradicated with application of topical mupirocin to the anterior nares. However, this therapy should be limited to patients with recurring MRSA infections and colonized hospital personnel to prevent the development of resistance.

The most common mode of *S. aureus* transmission is direct contact of body surface to body surface. The airborne route is less efficient but may occur in patients with *S. aureus* pneumonia or large burn wounds. Recently, it has been shown that colonized individuals with viral upper tract infections may shed *S. aureus* into the air. Transmission via indirect contact with inanimate objects such as instruments rarely occurs, but *S. aureus* can be detected on many surfaces in hospitals, including stethoscopes.

Strategies for the management of *S. aureus* and especially MRSA colonization or infection must focus on the type of spread. Epidemic outbreaks are successfully handled with prompt application of infection control measures. Application of precautions such as patient isolation, handwashing with antiseptic detergents or alcohol, and glove usage can interrupt the chain of transmission and control the outbreak. Institutions with repeated introduction of MRSA from the community or other facilities are unlikely to be able to eradicate this pathogen.

Treatment of systemic MRSA infections is limited to the use of glycopeptide antibiotics such as vancomycin and teicoplanin. Since vancomycin resistance can be transferred in vitro from enterococci to *S. aureus*, the spread of nontreatable vancomycin-resistant *S. aureus* (VRSA) is one of the grimmest potential scenarios for modern infection control. With the first detection of an intermediate vancomycin-resistant *S. aureus* isolate in Japan in the spring of 1997, this scenario became more of a reality. Implementation and stringent enforcement of isolation practices is the only hope of preventing the spread of these multiresistant strains.

References

Boyce JM, Jackson MM, Pugliese G, et al. Methicillin-resistant *Staphylococcus aureus* (MRSA): a briefing for acute care hospitals and nursing facilities. Infect Control Hosp Epidemiol 1994;15: 105–15.

Doebbeling BN, Breneman DL, Neu HC, et al. Elimination of *Staphylococcus aureus* nasal carriage in health care workers: analysis of six clinical trials with calcium mupirocin ointment. Clin Infect Dis 1993;17:466–74.

CHAPTER 31

ENTEROCOCCAL SPECIES

Michael B. Edmond, MD, MPH

Key Issue: Enterococci are important nosocomial pathogens because 1) they are the normal flora in the human gastrointestinal tract, 2) antimicrobial resistance allows for their survival in an environment with heavy antimicrobial usage, 3) they can survive in the environment for prolonged periods of time, and 4) contamination of the hands of health care workers coupled with poor handwashing compliance provides the potential for spread in the hospital.

Known Facts

- Enterococci are common hospital-acquired pathogens, accounting for 16% of nosocomial urinary tract infections, 12% of nosocomial wound infections, and 9% of nosocomial bloodstream infections.

- Over the past 3 decades, enterococci have acquired resistance to multiple classes of antimicrobials, including aminoglycosides (high level) and glycopeptides (vancomycin and teicoplanin).

- Transfer of vancomycin resistance from *E. faecalis* to *Staphylococcus aureus* has been accomplished in the laboratory, suggesting that the same could occur in nature.

- Vancomycin resistance in enterococci has accelerated over the past 5 to 10 years; currently, 15% of nosocomial enterococcal bloodstream isolates in the United States are resistant to vancomycin.

- *E. faecium* is much more commonly resistant to vancomycin than *E. faecalis* (50% versus 5%).

- Risk factors for acquisition of vancomycin-resistant enterococci (VRE) include prior use of antimicrobial agents (vancomycin, third-generation cephalosporins, antianaerobic drugs), length of hospital stay, and severity of illness.

- Risk factors for VRE bacteremia include neutropenia, gastrointestinal colonization, and hematologic malignancy.

Controversial Issues

- Treatment of VRE infections is problematic. Therapy should include drainage of localized infections, when possible. Quinupristin/dalfopristin may be clinically useful for the treatment of infections due to *E. faecium* but is inactive against *E. faecalis*.
- A few reports have described attempts to decolonize the gastrointestinal tract of VRE but results have been suboptimal.

Suggested Practice: For patients with VRE-infection or colonization:

- Place in private room or cohort with other VRE infected/colonized patients. Gloves should be worn on entering the patient's room.
- If contamination of the clothing or close contact with the patient is anticipated, a gown should be worn.
- Strict compliance with handwashing is critical—a medicated handwashing agent (e.g., chlorhexidine) or alcohol should be used.
- Noncritical items (e.g., stethoscopes, thermometers, etc.) should be left in the patient's room.
- Phenolic and quaternary ammonium disinfectants are active against VRE.

Summary: Enterococci are ubiquitous gram-positive cocci which are part of the normal flora of man and other animals. Infections caused by enterococci include urinary tract infections, abdominal-pelvic infections, wound (especially decubital and diabetic foot) infections, and endocarditis.

Over the past 3 decades, strains of enterococci have acquired resistance to essentially all available antimicrobial agents. The first reports of resistance to vancomycin were noted in the late 1980s. In general, antimicrobial resistance has been more problematic for *Enterococcus faecium* than *E. faecalis*.

In the United States, acquisition of VRE occurs primarily in the hospital. In Europe, many patients acquire the organism in the community. Community acquisition is felt to be due to the use of avoparcin, a glycopeptide antibiotic, as a supplement to animal feeds. Avoparcin is not used in the United States.

The prevalence of vancomycin resistance among the enterococci has been accelerating at an alarming rate. In 1989, less than 0.5% of enterococcal isolates from ICU and non-ICU settings were vancomycin resistant. In 1994, 9% of enterococci from patients in non-ICU settings and nearly 14% of isolates from ICUs were resistant to vancomycin.

Numerous case-control studies have evaluated risk factors for the development of colonization and/or infection with VRE. The most consistent factor for VRE colonization/infection has been prior treatment with vancomycin. However, a number of other antimicrobial agents, including ceftazidime, aminoglycosides, ciprofloxacin, aztreonam, and antianaerobic drugs have been identified as risk factors in at least one study. Other risk factors have included severity of illness, length of hospital stay, hematologic malignancy or bone marrow transplant, and mucositis. Colonization of the GI tract has been shown to be a risk factor for the development of VRE bacteremia. Several studies have documented that environmental contamination with VRE is common, especially when the patient has diarrhea.

To control VRE in the hospital setting, we recommend placing colonized/infected patients in a private room. Gloves should be worn on entering the patient's room, and strict attention should be paid to handwashing with chlorhexidine. In addition, there should be no sharing of noncritical items (i.e., BP cuffs, stethoscopes, etc., should remain in the patient's room). Housekeeping staff should wipe down all horizontal surfaces in VRE patient rooms daily.

In addition to infection control measures, controlling VRE requires prudent use of antibiotics, particularly vancomycin. Vancomycin should be avoided for routine surgical prophylaxis, empiric treatment of febrile neutropenia, treatment of a single positive blood culture for coagulase-negative staphylococci if contamination is likely, and primary treatment of antibiotic-associated colitis (metronidazole is preferred). In addition, vancomycin should not be continued empirically when cultures are negative for the beta-lactam-resistant gram-positive organisms. Vancomycin should not be used for selective gut decontamination or for routine prophylaxis of low-birth-weight infants, continuous ambulatory peritoneal dialysis patients, or intravascular catheters.

References

Edmond MB. Multidrug-resistant enterococci and the threat of vancomycin-resistant *Staphylococcus aureus*. In: Wenzel RP, editor. Prevention and Control of Nosocomial infections. 3rd ed. Baltimore: Williams and Wilkins; 1997:339–55.

Murray BE. Vancomycin-resistant enterococci. Am J Med 1997; 101:284–93.

CHAPTER 32

PNEUMOCOCCUS

Marc J. Struelens, MD, PhD

Key Issues: Separate waiting areas and hospital rooms or wards should be used for patients with acute chest infections and patients with immune deficiencies or chronic disease predisposing to invasive pneumococcal infection.

Known Facts
- Transmission occurs primarily via direct contact with infected patients with pneumonia or through large respiratory droplets.
- Invasive pneumococcal infections such as pneumonia, bacteremia, and meningitis carry a high mortality rate.
- Predisposing factors to invasive infection include very young and older age, splenectomy, malnutrition, alcoholism, diabetes, chronic cardiopulmonary disease, and immune deficiencies, including HIV infection.
- Resistance to major antibiotics, including penicillin, cephalosporins, and macrolides, is increasing worldwide.
- The importance of pneumococci as agents of endemic nosocomial infection is poorly defined.
- Small outbreaks with antibiotic-resistant strains occur in open wards in pediatric or adult patients with predisposing factors.

Suggested Practice
- Where possible, assign separate waiting and care areas (hospital rooms and wards) to patients with acute chest infection and patients at increased risk of invasive pneumococcal infection, including young infants, elderly patients, patients with splenectomy, diabetes, chronic lung and heart disease, and immune deficiency.
- Wear gloves and gowns when touching respiratory secretions from patients with acute respiratory tract infection. Discard

the gloves after use and wash or disinfect hands between patient contacts. Disinfect all respiratory care equipment, including mouthpieces, between uses for different patients.
- Administer polyvalent pneumococcal polysaccharide vaccine to adults and children above 2 years of age with risk factors for invasive pneumococcal disease.

Monitor the prevalence of penicillin and multidrug-resistant pneumococci from hospitalized patients with pneumonia. In case of increased prevalence, serotype strains to detect clusters of cross-infection. If an outbreak is documented, infected patients should be nursed in isolation and standard barrier precautions should be carefully observed.

Controversial Issue: The need for screening and subsequent attempt at eradication of *S. pneumoniae* carriage for controlling outbreaks with antibiotic-resistant strains is not well defined.

Summary: *Streptococcus pneumoniae* (a pneumococcus) is an elongated, gram-positive coccus that grows in pairs or short chains. It is catalase-negative, alpha-hemolytic, and is susceptible to optochin. It can be serotyped based on its capsular polysaccharides (80 serotypes). Its capsule is a major virulence factor that inhibits the alternate activation of the complement pathway and thereby blocks nonimmune phagocytosis. Polysaccharide-specific antibodies that appear approximately 7 days after infection or immunization greatly enhance phagocytosis and killing of the pneumococcus and confer serotype-specific protection. The pneumococcus releases toxins (pneumolysin) and proinflammatory cell-wall products upon cell lysis. It inhabits the pharynx (nose or throat) of asymptomatic carriers among 10 to 40% of healthy people, depending on age and season.

The commonest form of pneumococcal infection are acute otitis media and sinusitis. *S. pneumoniae* is the most frequent cause of community-acquired pneumonia and a common cause of bacteremia and meningitis. Factors predisposing to invasive pneumococcal disease include extremes of age (infants and elderly), splenectomy, malnutrition, alcoholism, diabetes mellitus, chronic cardiopulmonary disease, and immune deficiency. Incidence of pneumonia and bacteremia are increased 10- and 100-fold, respectively, among HIV-infected persons. Pneumococcal pneumonia, bacteremia, and meningitis carry a mortality rate ranging between 10 and 40%. Beta-lactams and macrolides are the main therapeutic agents. Resistance to both classes of drugs is increasing in many countries.

The importance of the pneumococcus as anosocomial pathogen is not well defined. Based on onset of symptoms and isolation more than 48 hours after admission, pneumococcal pneumonia has been considered hospital-acquired in up to 20 to 50% of cases in hospitalized adults with underlying disease or HIV infection.

Small nosocomial outbreaks (20 cases) due to penicillin-resistant or multidrug-resistant pneumococcal strains have been documented. These occurred mostly following admission of a patient with pneumococcal pneumonia to open wards where high-risk patients were managed together, including patients with cancer, elderly patients with chronic pulmonary disease, and children with measles and malnutrition. Carriers among patients and health care staff are uncommon and do not appear important in transmission. Contaminated equipment is rarely implicated, with a single report of transmission via an improperly disinfected ventilator mask.

Increased rates of isolation of antibiotic-resistant *S. pneumoniae* from cases of pneumonia in hospitalized patients should prompt an outbreak investigation. Serotyping should be done to delineate the pattern of transmission. Nursing the infected patients in isolation, careful handwashing and disinfection of respiratory equipment, and closing wards to new admissions may be required for outbreak control. Screening of carriers and eradication of carriage are more controversial control measures.

Prevention of nosocomial transmission can be achieved through immunization with polyvalent pneumococcal polysaccharide vaccine of adults and children above 2 years of age with predisposing factors. In addition, high-risk patients should be cared for in separate facilities (wards, waiting room, and outpatient clinic) from patients with acute chest infection.

References

Friedland IR, Klugman KP. Antibiotic-resistant pneumococcal disease in South-African children. Am J Dis Child 1992;146:920–3.

Millar MR, Brown NM, Tobin GW, Murphy PJ, Windsor ACM, Speller DCE. Outbreak of infection with penicillin-resistant *Streptococcus pneumoniae* in a hospital for the elderly. J Hosp Infect 1992;27:99–104.

CHAPTER 33

BACTERIAL ENTERIC PATHOGENS: SALMONELLA, SHIGELLA, ESCHERICHIA COLI, AND OTHERS

Sheikh Jalal Uddin, MSc, Olivier Vandenberg, MD,
Jean-Paul Butzler, MD, PhD

Key Issue: *Salmonella, Shigella, Escherichia coli, Clostridium difficile, Campylobacter, Yersinia enterocolitica, Vibrio cholerae,* and *Vibrio parahaemolyticus* are among the various agents which may cause acute gastrointestinal infections in patients and health care workers.

Known Facts

- Salmonellosis is the most commonly reported foodborne disease resulting from improperly handled animal and poultry products. Ninety-two percent of all cases are due to raw or partially cooked eggs but undercooked poultry, beef, and pork also are significant sources. Contamination may occur either during food processing by contact with animal products/feces, or during food preparation from food handlers. Chronic carriers of *Salmonella* pose a particular risk for transmitting this infection.

- In developing countries, nontyphoid *Salmonella* spp are increasingly important nosocomial pathogens, causing septicemia in children. Most of these *Salmonella* spp are resistant to multiple antibiotics. The dissemination of these resistant strains occurs from person to person.

- Shigellosis is one of the most common causes of gastroenteritis. Transmission is due to improper handwashing and inadequate toilet facilities and occurs via food items such as soups, salads, and sandwiches. After ingestion of a very low inoculum ($<10^2$) of shigella organisms, patients typically present with dysentery and fever. Patients are infectious during the acute infection and until the organism is no longer present in the feces.

- Transmission of enterotoxigenic *E. coli* (ETEC) occurs mainly by food and water. It very rarely occurs from person to person.

- Enterohemorrhagic *Escherichia coli* (EHEC), particularly *E. coli* serotype O157: H7, is the leading cause of hemorrhagic colitis and hemolytic uremic syndrome (HUS). Transmission is mainly via beef consumption. Sporadic person-to-person transmission has been reported.

- Enteropathogenic *Escherichia coli* (EPEC) is an infrequent cause of outbreaks of diarrhea in hospitalized infants.

- *Clostridium difficile* can be easily acquired during hospitalization, especially after antibiotic treatment. This pathogen easily spreads in the health care setting from infected patients to their environment. In hospitals, the isolation rate is high in toilets, bed pans, floors, and the hands of the personnel.

- In the last 10 years, *Campylobacter jejuni* has emerged as the most frequent cause of bacterial gastroenteritis. In developing countries, the disease is confined to young children. Immunity develops early in life through repeated exposure to infection. Transmission mainly occurs indirectly via contaminated food, milk, or water. Nosocomial spread within neonatal units has been observed on rare occasions. The putative causes of these outbreaks were an inadequately disinfected communal baby bath and an incubator that was not disinfected between babies.

- *Vibrio cholerae* is transmitted primarily via contaminated water and by the ingestion of contaminated shellfish. Person-to-person spread is uncommon. Hospital workers rarely contract the disease.

- *Vibrio parahaemolyticus* gastroenteritis is associated with the consumption of seafood. Symptoms can vary but patients usually present with nausea, vomiting, and cramps. Fever and chills sometimes can occur.

- *Yersinia enterocolitica* is a common cause of enterocolitis in children in developed countries. It is characterized by either watery or bloody diarrhea with abdominal pain and fever.

Improperly cooked pork and milk are the main sources of transmission. Nosocomial transmission occurs very rarely.

Controversial Issues

- Gastroenteritis caused by bacterial pathogens often may be confused with enteric infections caused by parasitic, fungal, or viral agents.
- The decision whether or not to use antibiotics or antimotility drugs is difficult in the absence of specific laboratory diagnosis of the bacterial pathogens.
- Indiscriminate treatment with antibiotic agents or antimotility drugs may create serious public health problems by encouraging the development of multidrug-resistant bacteria or chronic carriers.
- The incidence of acute gastroenteritis caused by enteric pathogens is greatly underestimated in many locations because of limited surveillance, limited laboratory facilities to diagnose the most common bacterial agents, or both.

Suggested Practice

- Most bacterial enteric pathogens are transmitted by direct contact. Effective handwashing practice is the most important measure to prevent transmission. Additional interventions include

  1. improvements in hygiene and socioeconomic conditions;
  2. safe water supply and sanitary disposal of fecally contaminated materials;
  3. thorough cooking of food; and
  4. segregation of ill persons.

- Food service personnel must be very careful about personal hygiene, working habits, and their health. All health care and food service personnel with an acute diarrheal illness should stop working until the diarrhea has resolved.
- Antibiotics should not be routinely used to prevent transmission. When antibiotics are used to treat patients, appropriate doses and duration of therapy should be used.

- All enteric bacteria isolated from nosocomial infections should be well characterized.

Summary: Bacterial enteric pathogens are a diverse group of intestinal bacteria representing different members of the gram-negative bacilli and a few of gram-positive bacteria. Among gram-negative bacteria, *Salmonella, Shigella, Vibrio, Escherichia coli, Campylobacter*, and *Yersinia* are the most common causes of gastroenteritis. *Clostridium, Staphylococcus aureus, Bacillus cereus,* and *Listeria monocytogenes* are known gram-positive enteric pathogens. Gastroenteritis caused by these different groups of bacteria is a leading cause of morbidity and mortality in developing countries. However, difficulty in identifying certain enteric pathogens in many laboratories leads to marked under-reporting.

The majority of the gastrointestinal pathogens are transmitted through the fecal-oral route. These pathogens can survive in soil, water, and food. Outbreaks are frequently related to ingestion of contaminated food or water and occur more frequently in developing countries. Improvements in hygiene and socioeconomic conditions can dramatically reduce the transmission of these organisms.

Recent studies from the developing world have emphasized the emerging importance of multidrug-resistant *Salmonella* spp as nosocomial pathogens in children. The clinical microbiologist should be responsible for the identification of all isolates of nosocomial infections and work effectively with all other members of the infection control committee to identify and control outbreaks.

References

DeMaio JD, Bishai WR. Food poisoning. In: Thomas Lamont, editor. Gastrointestinal infections: diagnosis and management. New York: Marcel Dekker Publisher; 1997. p. 87–123.

DuPont HL, Ribner BS. Infectious gastroenteritis. In: Bennett JB, Brachman PS, editors. Hospital infections. 4th ed. Philadelphia: Lippincott-Raven Publishers; 1998. p. 537–50.

CHAPTER 34

OTHER ENTEROBACTERIACEAE

Diane Franchi, MD, and Michael T. Wong, NM, MD

Key Issue: Enterobacteriaceae (other than enteropathogenic *Salmonella, Shigella,* and *E. coli*) are important nosocomial pathogens that play a significant role as etiologic agents of all nosocomial infections, especially of urinary tract infections, surgical site infections, and pneumonia.

Known Facts

- Colonization of the gastrointestinal tract and/or the oropharynx of hospitalized patients with Enterobacteriaceae (whether endogenous or exogenously acquired) increases the risk for nosocomial infections.
- Modes of transmission of Enterobacteriaceae in the hospital setting include person-to-person spread (via the hands of health care workers) and, to a lesser degree, environmental contamination, especially of moist surfaces.
- The emergence of multiresistant Enterobacteriaceae containing extended spectrum beta-lactamases and cephalosporinases is becoming a worldwide problem.
- Simple soap and water handwashing will remove almost all transient gram-negative rods in 10 seconds.

Controversial Issues

- Ventilated patients whose stomach pH remains below 4.0 are more likely to become colonized with Enterobacteriaceae in the gastrointestinal tract, the oropharynx, and the trachea if they receive antacids or histamine receptor (H_2) blockers for stress ulcer prophylaxis rather than sucralfate. Because of higher rates of colonization, those receiving antacids or H_2 blockers are at increased risk for nosocomial pneumonia.

- Selective decontamination of the oropharynx and gastro-intestinal tract of ventilated patients with nonabsorbable antibiotics may be useful in controlling an outbreak of multiresistant Enterobacteriaceae when more conventional infection control strategies fail.

Suggested Practice

Prevention of Transmission.
  A. Susceptible Strains
    1. Strict handwashing as detailed in Chapter 2.
    2. Identification and elimination of environmental sources.
  B. Multiresistant Strains
    1. All measures detailed above for susceptible strains.
    2. Isolation of colonized or infected patients.
    3. Contact precautions: gowns, gloves, and single-use or dedicated equipment.
    4. Decrease nurse-to-patient ratio, when possible.
    5. Cohort patients and health care providers if an outbreak (two or more infections) occurs.

Prevention of the Evolution of Colonization with Enterobacteriaceae to Infection.
    1. Discontinue indwelling urinary catheters, nasogastric tubes, and endotracheal tubes as soon as possible.
    2. Routine rotation of intravenous catheter sites (peripheral and central).

For specific recommendations concerning enteropathogenic Enterobacteriaceae, bladder catheterization, ventilators, and preoperative patient care, see the appropriate chapter.

Summary: Enterobacteriaceae comprise a family of gram-negative bacilli that are facultative anaerobes. The family Enterobacteriaceae contains genera such as *Citrobacter, Enterobacter, Escherichia, Klebsiella, Proteus, Salmonella, Serratia,* and

Shigella. The discussion and guidelines in this chapter do not include those for the enteric pathogens *Salmonella, Shigella,* and enterpathogenic *E. coli.*

Major reservoirs of Enterobacteriaceae are water, soil, and the human gastrointestinal tract. Many people carry Enterobacteriaceae as part of their oropharyngeal flora even before admission to the hospital. This can be as high as 60% in alcoholics. Colonization is usually with a small number of colonies but may increase with selective antibiotic pressure. Colonization in the hospital is usually by indirect spread via the hands of health care workers or via contaminated equipment and supplies. Risk for nosocomial infection increases dramatically once colonization of a patient is established.

References

Doebbeling BN, Stanley GL, Sheetz CT, et al. Comparative efficacy of alternative handwashing agents in reducing nosocomial infection in intensive care units. N Engl J Med 1992;327:88–93.

Hariharan R, Weinstein RA. Enterobacteriaceae. In: Mayhall CG, editor. Hospital epidemiology and infection control. Baltimore: Williams and Wilkins Publishers; 1996. p. 345–66.

Soulier A, Barbut F, Ollivier JC, et al. Decreased transmission of Enterobacteriaceae with extended-spectrum β-lactamases in an intensive care unit by nursing reorganization. J Hosp Infect 1995; 31:89–97.

CHAPTER 35

PSEUDOMONAS AERUGINOSA

Richard P. Wenzel, MD, MSc

Key Issue: *Pseudomonas aeruginosa*, a ubiquitous organism, is increasingly important as a cause of serious nosocomial infections.

Known Facts: *Pseudomonas aeruginosa* is an aerobic gram-negative rod found in water and soil and uncommonly as normal flora in humans. It is commonly found in the environment of hospitals, especially in the presence of moisture. It is the sixth leading cause of nosocomial bloodstream infection in many US hospitals, and often it is resistant to many commonly used antibiotics. This organism is virulent but it is also a major cause of infection in neutropenic patients.

Controversial Issues: There are still limited data on the epidemiology of infections caused by *Pseudomonas aeruginosa*. Particularly controversial is the mode of transmission via the hands of medical personnel.

Suggested Practice: There should be no standing water or moisture from water or medical solutions in a hospital. When found, they should be eliminated to avoid a reservoir of *Pseudomonas aeruginosa*. Additionally, whenever there is a cluster of infections caused by this organism, a careful review of all medical solutions used in the environment must be carried out in seeking the reservoir.

Summary: Outbreaks of infections caused by *Pseudomonas aeruginosa* have been traced to contaminated water for injection, contaminated tracheal irrigant solutions, mouthwash, inadequately disinfected endoscopes, and tap water.

In studies of nosocomial bloodstream infection, *Pseudomonas aeruginosa* as the offending organism has been shown to be an independent predictor of mortality.

References

Morris AJ, Wenzel RP. Epidemiology of infection due to *Pseudomonas aeruginosa*. Rev Infect Dis 1984;6:S627–42.

Widmer AF, Wenzel RP, Trilla A, et al. Outbreak of *Pseudomonas aeruginosa* infections in a surgical intensive care unit: probable transmission via hands of a health care worker. Clin Infect Dis 1993;16:372–6.

CHAPTER 36

HELICOBACTER PYLORI

Jeanne-Marie Devaster, MD,
Patience Mandisodza, MSc, and Anne Dediste, MD

Key Issue: *Helicobacter pylori* is the commonest chronic bacterial infection in humans, colonizing approximately 60% of the world's population.

Known Facts

- *H. pylori* is implicated as a causal factor in duodenal ulcer disease, gastric ulcer disease, and in the development of gastric cancers.
- Most persons infected with *H. pylori* are asymptomatic.
- In developing countries, contamination is maximal in childhood, the prevalence of *H. pylori* infection being as high as 50% by the age of 5 years.
- Treatment is strongly recommended in peptic ulcer disease and low-grade gastric mucosa-associated lymphoid tissue (MALT) lymphoma when *H. pylori* is present.
- Iatrogenic transmission of *H. pylori* by upper gastrointestinal endoscopy has been documented and is probably underestimated due to the need of both long-term follow-up in asymptomatic patients and invasive procedures.
- *H. pylori* shows sensitivity to the most commonly used high level disinfectants and, therefore, iatrogenic inoculation of the bacterium by endoscopy is unlikely to occur if appropriate disinfection procedures are strictly adopted.

Controversial Issues

- The human stomach is thought to be the natural reservoir of *H. pylori* and its spread seems to occur mainly by person-to-person transmission, either by fecal-oral or oral-oral routes.
- There is no evidence that asymptomatic patients should be treated.

- In practice in developing countries, presumptive treatment seems to be followed in most of the cases by recurrence.
- In the future, active or passive immunization will be the solution.

Suggested Practice

- Wearing of gloves during potential contaminating procedures such as endoscopy, exposure to patients' secretions (feces, vomitus, gastric aspirates), and handling of potentially contaminated objects (syringes, biopsy forceps, pH electrodes).
- Strict adherence to disinfection procedures of gastrointestinal endoscopes between each patients:
  - Adequate washing of instruments before disinfection
  - Use of appropriate disinfectant
  - Respect of immersion time of endoscopes in disinfectant
  - Biopsy forceps and devices breaching the gastric mucosa should be considered as critical items and therefore sterilized.

Summary: Overwhelming evidence now confirms that *H. pylori* is a worldwide infection and plays an etiologic role in the development of chronic superficial gastritis and peptic ulcer disease. *H. pylori* infection is also strongly associated with gastric adenocarcinoma and MALT lymphomas. The bacterium infects 25 to 50% of the general population in developed countries while in most developing countries, infection rates can be as high as 80 to 90%, especially in the case of poor socioeconomic and sanitary conditions. Most infected persons tend to be asymptomatic, with only a minority developing peptic ulceration and even fewer gastric cancer.

   The exact mode of transmission and spread of *H. pylori* infection in the community are still unclear. No substantial reservoir of *H. pylori* has been identified, besides the human stomach, and spread is believed to occur by person-to-person transmission. Several arguments favoring both fecal-oral and oral-oral means have been substantiated by different studies. The presence of

H. pylori in feces, although rarely detected, and epidemiological evidence in developing countries that implicates feces or fecal contamination as a risk factor, support the fecal-oral route. In favor of the oral-oral transmission is the presence of the bacterium in gastric juice, dental plaque, and saliva. Supporting this way of transmission, feeding of premasticated food by mothers to their infants in Africa has been identified as a risk factor for *H. pylori* infection in young children. It is possible that both routes of transmission exist although newer potential reservoirs of *H. pylori* have now been identified, such as nonhuman primates, cats, flies, and environmental sources such as water.

The third and least common route of *H. pylori* transmission is iatrogenic inoculation of strains from one patient to another through a contaminated endoscope. Fiberoptic endoscopic examination of the gastrointestinal tract is known to result in iatrogenic transmission of infectious agents, such as *Salmonella* spp, *Pseudomonas* spp, *Acinetobacter* spp. Since the proportion of individuals positive for *H. pylori* consists of about half the world's population, the potential for endoscopic contamination with *H. pylori* and further iatrogenic transmission is high. It is further complicated by the complex internal design of endoscopes and the difficulty of decontamination (metal and plastic components, and fiberoptic glass). Several studies have shown that contamination of endoscopes and biopsy forceps occurs readily after endoscopic examination of *H. pylori*-positive patients. Iatrogenic proof of transmission of the bacterium has been estimated at about 4/1000 endoscopies when the infection rate in the endoscoped population is about 60%. Traditional cleaning and alcohol rinsing of endoscopic equipment has been proven insufficient to eliminate endoscope/biopsy forceps contamination.

A number of guidelines specific to the processing of endoscopes have been published. Endoscopes are classified as semicritical items according to Spaulding, and should at least receive high-level disinfection. Accessories, such as biopsy forceps that breach the mucosa, are considered as critical devices and therefore must be mechanically cleaned and then sterilized after each use. Disinfection of medical equipment is detailed in Chapter 5, and only a few points related to upper gastrointestinal endoscopy will be described here:

- Every endoscopic procedure should be performed with a clean, disinfected endoscope.
- All endoscopic units must have written guidelines for decontamination.
- As the status of the patient is often not known, all patients should be considered as potentially contaminated and thus treated with the same procedure.
- Manual brushing of the endoscope surface, valves, all internal channels (they should be thoroughly flushed with water and detergent), and endoscopic accessories (biopsy forceps, pH electrodes), has to be done immediately after each patient to prevent drying of secretions. This step is mandatory before the disinfection process (even if an automated washer is used). It is accomplished with water, mechanical action, and suitable detergents or enzymatic products.
- Disinfection: The endoscope should be immersed in 2% glutaraldehyde or other equivalent chemical disinfectant. All channels must be filled with the disinfectant. The 20-minute exposure time is recommended to achieve high-level disinfection. However, if impracticable due to turnover pressure and when *Mycobacterium tuberculosis* is not suspected, 10 to 20 minutes' time is usually considered acceptable (10 minutes being the minimum).
- Rinsing of the instruments with preferably sterile water internally and externally to remove all traces of disinfectant, and remembering that glutaraldehyde and most chemical disinfectants have serious side effects are necessary. If tap water is used, rinsing the external surface as well as all channels with 70% alcohol and thoroughly drying them by compressed air is recommended.

- In all cases, drying channels with compressed air will prevent growth of bacteria in a moist environment.
- Storage of the equipment should be done with care, and it is best to hang the endoscopes to drain any excess water in channels (especially in areas where forced air drying is not possible).

In conclusion, thorough cleaning and disinfection schedules are adequate to prevent iatrogenic transmission of common bacterial (including *H. pylori*) and viral infections from one patient to the next one through contaminated endoscopes. However, much more understanding of the exact ways of transmission of *H. pylori* in the community is needed to develop specific guidelines to limit the spread of the infection in the general population.

References

Dunn BE, Cohen H, Blaser MJ. Helicobacter pylori. Clin Microbiol Rev 1997;10:720–41.

Martin MA, Reichelderfer M. APIC guideline for infection prevention and control in flexible endoscopy. Am J Infect Control 1994; 22:19–38.

CHAPTER 37

FUNGI

Sergio B. Wey, MD

Key Issue: The incidence of nosocomial fungal infections has increased in recent years.

Known Facts

- *Candida* spp has been found to be the fourth most commonly isolated infective agent in the blood, following *S. aureus*, *S. epidermidis*, and *Enterococcus*.
- The incidence of candidemia is higher in critical care units than in other parts of the hospital.
- Approximately two-thirds of primary fungemias are associated with the use of central venous catheters and the same proportion are encountered in intensive care units (ICUs).
- Most cases of nosocomial fungemia found in intensive care unit patients are not associated with recognized immune defense defects.
- Fungemia is associated with a high short-term mortality rate. The crude mortality exceeds 55% and attributable mortality is approximately 38%.
- Recent prospective trials have identified persistence of *Candida* species in repetitive cultures at various sites as an essential, if not necessary, precursor for fungemia.
- Fungi can also cause important infections in long-term intravascular catheters.
- It is already well documented that *Candida* infections, even candidemia, can be transmitted on the hands of colonized health care personnel.
- The evidence for cross-infection by *Candida*, particularly in ICUs, has increased in the literature.
- The incidence of non-*albicans Candida* infections are increasing. They tend to be more resistant to azoles than *C. albicans* strains.

- Positive blood cultures with *Candida* require the immediate removal of all central venous catheters.

Controversial Issues

- The role of susceptibility testing as a guide to selecting appropriate therapy for all of these infections is as yet incompletely defined.
- Use of antibiotic prophylaxis for patients requiring prolonged intensive care unit residence who are colonized with *Candida*, based on the frequency with which such patients progress to fungemia.
- Whether fluconazole is a safe alternative for treatment of candidemia, mainly in infections by non-*albicans* species.

Suggested Practice

- Proper use of antibiotics and invasive procedures.
- Define therapy based on yeast identification.

Summary: *Candida* and *Aspergillus* are responsible for the vast majority of hospital-acquired fungal infections. However, several other species such as *Trichosporon* and *Fusarium* can cause infection in debilitated hospitalized patients.

Several institutions have reported an increased rate of nosocomial fungal infections. Bloodstream infections are one of the most serious hospital-acquired infections. Many are caused by the use of vascular catheters.

From January 1980 to December 1990, 30,477 fungal isolates causing nosocomial infections were reported from 180 hospitals participating in the National Nosocomial Infections Surveillance (NNIS) system. The nosocomial fungal infection rate at these facilities increased from 2.0 infections per 1000 patients discharged in 1980 to 3.8 in 1990; cases of nosocomial fungemia rose from 1.0 to 4.9. The proportion of nosocomial infections, reported by all hospitals, that are due to fungal pathogens (from all major sites of infection) rose from 6% in 1980 to 10.4% in 1990, and the proportion due to nosocomial bloodstream infection increased from 5.4% to 9.9%. The proportion of bloodstream infections due to fungal pathogens varied depending on patient care characteristics. Patients who had a central intravascular catheter were more than three times as likely to have a fungus isolated as were patients with bloodstream infections that did not have catheters ($p < .001$). *Candida* species accounted for 72% of these isolates.

Fungemia is associated with a high short-term mortality rate. The crude mortality exceeds 55%. The attributable mortality due to nosocomial candidemia has been estimated as 38%. Nosocomial bloodstream infections caused by *Candida* spp or *Pseudomonas* spp are independent predictors of death. An NNIS analysis showed that patients with fungemia were more likely to die during hospitalization (29%) than were patients with bloodstream infections due to nonfungal pathogens (17%; relative risk = 1.8%; 95% confidence interval = 1.7 to 1.9; $p < .001$).

Predisposing factors for fungal infections are well known and include leukemia, lymphoma, bone marrow or solid organ transplant, diabetes, severe burns, premature birth, chemotherapy, immunosuppressive drugs, broad-spectrum antibiotics, indwelling catheters, and prolonged hospitalization. Total parenteral nutrition is considered an important risk factor. Most cases of nosocomial fungemia found in intensive care unit patients were not associated with recognized immune defense defects. Independent risk factors for nosocomial fungemia include prior treatment with multiple antibiotics, prior Hickman catheterization, isolation of *Candida* species from sites other than the blood, prior hemodialysis, azotemia, recent major abdominal surgery, prolonged hospital stay, severity of acute illness, candiduria, large burns, and prematurity. It is likely that the administration of broad-spectrum antibiotics plays a role in eradicating endogenous competing flora and promoting overgrowth of yeast. One study showed that 38% of ICU patients who had been colonized by *Candida* developed a candida infection. Recent prospective trials have identified persistence of *Candida* species in repetitive cultures from various sites as an essential, if not necessary, precursor for fungemia.

It has been well documented that the transmission of *Candida* can occur via the hands of colonized health care personnel. There have been several outbreaks of candidemia in different populations of patients that could be tracked to the presence of the agent in the hands of hospital personnel, particularly in ICUs. Approximately 40% of health care workers in surgical intensive care units have *Candida* colonization of their hands.

There is a strong relationship between *Candida parapsilosis* fungemia or systemic infection and hyperalimentation using intravascular devices. The capability of *C. parapsilosis* isolates to proliferate and produce large amounts of slime in glucose-containing solutions may help to explain their ability to adhere to plastic material and cause catheter-related fungemia.

The incidence of the different species of *Candida* varies according to hospital and region. In the US, there has been great variation in the proportion of cases due to *C. albicans* compared to those due to non-*albicans* species. Recent data from six university hospitals in Brazil show that 77% of the yeast isolated in blood cultures were nonalbicans. Azoles were rarely used in these hospitals, which suggests selective pressure was not responsible.

As is the case with antibacterial agents, the increasing use of antifungal agents has led to the development of antifungal resistance, the most clinically important of which is the resistance of *Candida* to fluconazole. Fluconazole resistance for ICU patients happens with a shift away from susceptible species, such as *C. albicans* and *C. parapsilosis*, toward more resistant species such as *C. glabrata* and *C. krusei*. The role of susceptibility testing as a guide to selecting appropriate therapy for these infections is as yet incompletely defined but testing for resistance to fluconazole may soon be available for clinical use.

Candida spp can be a cause of suppurative peripheral thrombophlebitis. The pathogenesis of this infection appears to be the result of preceding candidal colonization of the skin and inadequate intravenous site care in susceptible patients, permitting candidal infection of the catheter wound and progression to the venous wall. Additionally, candidemia from other sites could cause colonization of the catheter with subsequent candidal thrombophlebitis. Fungal thrombophlebitis is a major risk for those with indwelling intravascular catheters. The main infection control measures for the prevention of fungal colonization of indwelling intravascular catheters are similar to those recommended for bacterial infections and have been outlined elsewhere. Candidal peripheral thrombophlebitis can be prevented by vigorous skin preparation, meticulous site care, and routine rotation of intravenous catheter sites every 48 to 72 hours. Other infection control measures to prevent peripheral candidal thrombophlebitis include limiting the spectrum and duration of antimicrobial therapy to specific culture-defined organisms for short intervals. Removal of the catheter is indicated in the following situations: documented *Candida* or fungal catheter-associated infection, purulent tunnel infection, or breakthrough bacteremia after the third day of appropriate intravenous antimicrobial therapy.

The efficacy of antifungal prophylaxis for patients colonized with *Candida* is unknown, and clinical trials are needed.

Reference

Beck-Sagué CM, Jarvis R, and the National Nosocomial Infections Surveillance System. Secular trends in the epidemiology of nosocomial fungal infections in the United States, 1980–1990. J Infect Dis 1993;167:1247–51.

CHAPTER 38

VIRUSES

C. M. A. Swanink, MD, PhD, and Andreas Voss, MD, PhD

Key Issue: Viral infections are common in the community and can cause a variety of symptoms.

Known Facts

- Diagnosis is based on antigen detection, antibody response, electron microscopy, virus isolation, or polymerase chain reaction, which may be laborious and/or time-consuming. Based on the route of transmission, viral infections can be classified into four categories:
  1. gastrointestinal infection (vomiting and diarrhea)
  2. respiratory tract infection (droplet infection)
  3. exanthematous disease (skin lesions, vesicles)
  4. bloodborne infection

Gastrointestinal Infection. Gastrointestinal infections are caused by several viruses that can be found in feces, such as: enteroviruses (polioviruses, coxsackieviruses A and B, echoviruses), adenoviruses, rotaviruses, astroviruses, caliciviruses (e.g., Norwalk virus, hepatitis E virus), small round viruses (SRV), small round structured viruses (SRSV), coronaviruses, and hepatitis A virus. Some of these are also found in respiratory secretions (enteroviruses, adenoviruses, coronaviruses) and may cause symptoms of an upper respiratory tract infection. Outbreaks are common in children in day care centers, and elderly people in nursing homes.

- Route of transmission is predominantly fecal-oral, often via contaminated hands. Thus, infection control strategies should focus on contact with fecally contaminated items and include gowns, gloves, and handwashing (see Table 38.1). In general, masks are not advised but should be worn during close contacts or high-risk procedures (e.g., bronchial toilet).

- Most infections are mild, self-limiting, and do not require any specific therapy.
- Vaccination is available for polioviruses, hepatitis A, hepatitis B, varicella, influenza, measles, mumps, rubella, and rabies.

Respiratory Tract Infection. Symptoms of respiratory tract infections may vary from common cold to life-threatening pneumonia or pneumonitis. Severity of the clinical symptoms is largely dependent on host defenses. Cytomegalovirus, for example, can cause severe pneumonitis in the immunocompromised host whereas most infections are subclinical in the immunocompetent host. Viruses that cause respiratory tract infections include influenza viruses, parainfluenza viruses, respiratory syncytial virus, adenoviruses, enteroviruses, rhinoviruses, and coronaviruses. Many other viruses can be found in respiratory secretions, such as cytomegalovirus (CMV), Epstein-Barr virus (EBV), herpes simplex virus (HSV), human herpes virus type 6 (HHV-6), measles, mumps, human parvovirus B19, rabies virus, rubella virus, poxviruses, and varicella-zoster virus (VZV).

- Route of transmission is via airborne spread or via contaminated hands. Infection control measures should be aimed at aerosol transmission and direct contact and may include isolation, masks, gowns, gloves, and handwashing.
- Influenza virus vaccination should be considered for high-risk patients. Amantadine may be useful in epidemic influenza A situations if given within 48 hours after exposure.
- Antiviral therapy is required in disseminated HSV infection and VZV infection in the immunocompromised patients and neonates because mortality is high in these patients.
- Neonates and susceptible immunocompromised adults who had contact with chickenpox or shingles should be given a dose of varicella-zoster immune globulin (VZIG) within 3 days after exposure. Varicella-zoster immune globulin may not prevent infection but it may reduce the severity of infection.

- In case of exposure to rabies virus, injection of human rabies immune globulin (HRIG) in the exposure site within 24 hours is recommended, followed by vaccination.
- A combined vaccine for mumps, measles, and rubella (MMR) should be given to children at the age of 12 to 18 months.

Exanthematous Disease. Many viral infections can cause exanthema, vesicles, or other skin lesions. The most common viruses are enteroviruses, herpes simplex virus (HSV), human herpes virus type 6 (HHV-6), varicella-zoster virus (VZV), measles, human parvovirus B19, and rubella virus.

- Route of transmission is via respiratory secretions (all) and skin lesions (HSV, VZV, coxsackievirus A). Infection control measures are listed in Table 38.1.
- Antiviral therapy is available for HSV and VZV.
- Vaccines for mumps, measles, and rubella are normally live attenuated vaccines and should not be given to severely immunocompromised patients.
- Less frequently occurring viruses that can cause nosocomial infections include those causing hemorrhagic fevers such as arenaviruses (Lassa, Machupo, Junin), and *Filoviruses* (Marburg and Ebola). These viruses require strict isolation because they are transmitted by blood and body fluids (see bloodborne infections). Several arboviruses, such as dengue and yellow fever, and rickettsiae may cause hemorrhagic skin lesions but they are vectorborne, and person-to-person transmission does not occur.
- Hantaviruses may cause hemorrhagic fever with renal syndrome but may also cause a pulmonary syndrome with rapid respiratory failure and cardiogenic shock. Hantaviruses are transmitted via infected rodent excreta. Person-to-person transmission does not occur; therefore, no preventive measures are required.

Bloodborne Infection. Hepatitis B virus (HBV), hepatitis C virus (HCV), human T-cell leukemia/lymphoma virus (HTLV),

Table 38.1

Virus/Infection	Infective Material	Isolation/ Precautions	Gown	Gloves	Mask	Single Room	Prevention/ Postexposure Prophylaxis
Adenovirus	resp. secretions, feces	contact	(+)	+	(+)	–	
AIDS/HIV	blood, body fluids	universal	–	+	–	–	(+) eye protection, + triple therapy
Astrovirus	feces	enteric	(+)	+	–	–	
Calicivirus	feces	enteric	(+)	+	–	–	
Coronavirus	resp. secretions, feces	contact	(+)	+	(+)	–	
Coxsackie A virus (hand-foot-mouth disease, herpangina)	resp. secretions, feces, lesions, secretions	contact	(+)	+	(+)	–	
Cytomegalovirus	resp. secretions, urine, breast milk	body fluids	–	+	(–)	–	+ avoid contact during pregnancy (+) ganciclovir (anti-CMV-immune globulin)
Dengue virus	blood	universal	–	+	–	–	+ avoid mosquito exposure, repellents
Enterovirus	resp. secretions, feces	contact	(+)	+	(–)	–	
Hantavirus (e.g., Puumala)	rodent excreta	none	–	–	–	–	
Hemorrhagic fever (Ebola, Marburg, Lassa)	blood, body fluids	strict	+	+	+	+	(+) eye protection, + ribavirin may be useful for Lassa fever
Hepatitis A and E viruses	feces	enteric	(+)	+	–	–	+ vaccination and immune globulin for HAV

Table 38.1 continued

Virus/Infection	Infective Material	Isolation/Precautions	Gown	Gloves	Mask	Single room	Prevention/Postexposure prophylaxis
Hepatitis B and D viruses	blood, body fluids	universal	–	+	–	–	(+) eye protection, + vaccination and HBIG
Hepatitis C, F, G viruses	blood, body fluids (?)	universal	–	+	–	–	(+) eye protection, (–) interferon
Herpes simplex virus (localized)	lesions, secretions	drainage, lesions, secretions	–	+	–	–	(+) acyclovir
Herpes simplex virus (disseminated)	lesions, secretions, resp. secretions	contact	+	+	(–)	+	(+) acyclovir
Herpes zoster virus (localized)	lesions, secretions	drainage, lesions, secretions	–	+	–	(–)	(+) VZIG
Herpes zoster virus (disseminated, varicella)	lesions, secretions, resp. secretions	strict	+	+	+	+	(+) vaccination, VZIG
HIV/HTLV	blood, body fluids	universal	–	+	–	–	(+) eye protection, + triple therapy
Influenza virus	resp. secretions	respiratory	–	(+)	(+)	+	(+) vaccination, amantadine
Measles	resp. secretions	respiratory	–	(–)	(+)	(–)	+ vaccination (MMR)
Mumps	resp. secretions	respiratory	–	(–)	(+)	(–)	+ vaccination (MMR)

Table 38.1 continued

Virus/Infection	Infective Material	Isolation/Precautions	Gown	Gloves	Mask	Single room	Prevention/Postexposure prophylaxis
Parainfluenza virus	resp. secretions	contact	–	(+)	(+)	–	
Parvovirus B19	resp. secretions, blood	contact	–	+	(+)	–	+ avoid contact during pregnancy
Poliovirus	resp. secretions, feces	enteric	(+)	+	(–)	–	+ vaccination
Rabies virus	resp. secretions	respiratory	(+)	+	(+)	–	+ HRIG at exposure site, vaccination
RSV bronchiolitis	resp. secretions	contact	+	+	(–)	+	+ single room only in children
Rotavirus	feces, resp. secretions	contact	+	+	(+)	–	+ hand disinfection (!)
Rubella virus	resp. secretions	contact	+	+	+	+	+ avoid contact during pregnancy, vaccination (MMR)
Small round virus (SRV, SRSV)	feces	contact	(+)	+	–	–	
Varicella	resp. secretions, lesions	strict	+	+	+	+	(+) vaccination, VZIG
Yellow fever	blood	–	–	+	–	–	+ avoid mosquito exposure, vaccination

+ = advised; (+) = only during high-risk procedures (e.g., bronchial toilet, soiling), high-risk patients, or close contact; (–) = questionable, probably not necessary; – = not necessary

human immunodeficiency virus (HIV), and viral hemorrhagic fevers (VHF) (e.g., Lassa, Marburg, Ebola) are examples of bloodborne infections. Other viral infections that can be transmitted by blood are CMV, EBV, and HHV-6 because these viruses persist in leukocytes.

- Routes of transmission are blood and body fluids, including breast milk. The risk of infection after a needlestick is 5 to 40% for HBV, 1 to 10% for HCV, and <0.5% for HIV. For VHF, exact data on transmission after needlestick accidents are missing, but it is known that high concentration of viruses are found in blood during the febrile period.
- Universal precautions should be taken when handling blood in all patients.
- Effective postexposure prophylaxis for HBV consists of passive immunization with hepatitis B immune globulin (HBIG) followed by active immunization with recombinant hepatitis B vaccine.
- Interferon prophylaxis after exposure to HCV is questionable.
- Triple therapy with a combination of a protease inhibitor and two reverse transcriptase inhibitors is probably useful as HIV postexposure prophylaxis.
- Ribavirin is an effective treatment for Lassa fever and may be useful as prophylaxis for Lassa fever.

References

Benenson AS, editor. Control of communicable diseases manual. 5th ed. Washington: American Public Health Association; 1995.

Fields DN, Knipe DM, Howley PM, editors. Fields virology. 3rd ed. Philadelphia: Lippincott-Raven Publishers; 1995.

Hu DJ, Kane MA, Heymann DL. Transmission of HIV, hepatitis B virus, and other bloodborne pathogens in health care settings: a review of risk factors and guidelines for prevention. World Health Organization. Bull World Health Organ 1991;69:623–30.

Weber DJ, Rutala WA, Hamilton H. Prevention and control of varicella zoster infections in health care facilities. Infect Control Hosp Epidemiol 1996;17:694–705.

CHAPTER 39

Infection Hazards of Human Cadavers

T. D. Healing, MSc, PhD,
P. Hoffman, BSc, and S. E. J. Young, FRCP

Key Issue: Cadavers may pose hazards to those handling them. None of the organisms that caused mass death in the past (e.g., plague, cholera, typhoid, tuberculosis, anthrax, or smallpox) is likely to survive long in burials. The recently dead may have been infected by a wide range of pathogens, with those presenting particular risks, including tuberculosis, streptococcal infection, gastrointestinal organisms, the agents causing transmissible spongiform encephalopathies (e.g., Creutzfeldt-Jakob disease), hepatitis B and C, HIV infection, hemorrhagic fever viruses, and possibly meningitis and septicemia (especially meningococcal).

Known Facts

- Long-buried bodes reduced to skeletons are not a hazard.
- Soft tissues remaining on a cadaver could present a risk.
- A possible hazard in old burials is anthrax, which can form resistant spores. This is unlikely; furthermore, humans are not very susceptible to this type of infection.
- Most of the microorganisms that people die of do not survive for long after their host dies.

Controversial Issues

- There have been worries that smallpox might survive in buried bodies. There is no good evidence that it happens. However, if a risk from this disease is expected, exhumations should be undertaken by people who have been vaccinated against smallpox in the past and who have a good scar. People should not be vaccinated against smallpox especially to deal with this hazard. The risks of smallpox vaccination greatly outweigh the theoretical risk of the virus surviving in cadavers.

Suggested Practice: Whether dealing with old burials or with the recently dead, regardless of which infectious agents may be present, the risk of acquiring infection can be greatly reduced by the following:

- Covering cuts or lesions with waterproof dressings
- Careful cleansing of any injuries sustained during procedures
- Good personal hygiene
- The use of appropriate protective clothing (Table 39.1)

Summary: Most people have little to do with the dead although they may at some time in their lives need to deal with the cadavers of relatives or friends during burial rituals. Others have jobs that regularly bring them into contact with cadavers, exposing them to the risk of acquiring infections. These include doctors (especially pathologists), nurses, mortuary attendants, forensic scientists, embalmers, funeral directors, priests, members of the emergency services, or others who routinely prepare bodies for the funeral or who perform funeral rites.

In most circumstances, the diseased living are a much greater hazard than are the dead, including those who have died of infectious diseases. While a person is alive, invading pathogens can multiply and are readily transmitted. The patient may be a continuing source of infection. Once the host is dead, most microorganisms stop multiplying and die rapidly.

The Recently Dead. The diseases and organisms which may pose particular risks vary in different parts of the world but include tuberculosis, streptococcal infection, gastrointestinal organisms, Creutzfeldt-Jakob disease (CJD), hepatitis and HIV infection, a number of viral infections (particularly viral hemorrhagic fevers such as Lassa or Ebola), and possibly meningitis and septicemia (especially meningococcal) (Table 39.2). In general, as with old burials, the use of appropriate protective clothing will greatly reduce the risk of acquiring infection but some additional precautions may be advisable for particular infections.

Tuberculosis. Opening cadavers of individuals infected with tuberculosis is dangerous, and workers in morbid anatomy, pathologists, mortuary technicians, and medical students have a high rate of tuberculin conversion. BCG vaccination is advised for such individuals.

Meningitis and Septicemia.

• Meningitis can be caused by a wide range of organisms but

Table 39.1 Protective Clothing

Hands

Examination gloves (latex). For handling hazardous material. Wear whenever handling bodies. Should be worn once only and then discarded. Always wash hands after use. Provide short-term (10-minute) protection against formaldehyde.

Chemically protective gloves (nitrile). Worn over examination gloves to protect from longer-term exposure to chemical hazards (e.g., formaldehyde).

Respiratory Protection

Filter masks. Filter mask to EN 149 for specific hazards (e.g., lead dust, fungal spores, and other aerosols).

Cloth surgical masks. These provide little protection and may give a false sense of security but are better than nothing.

Splash Protection

Face: visor. Protection against hazardous splashes to eyes, nose, and mouth (also mechanical protection).

Body: apron. Where splashing to body may occur (hygienic preparation, embalming, collection of traumatized bodies, postmortem examinations).

Feet: rubber boots. In wet situations (mortuaries, embalming rooms, collecting severe multiple trauma cases).

Whole-Body Protection

Gowns/coats. To protect clothing against splashing.

Coverall with hood. To protect clothes and hair from impregnation with dusts, spores, etc.

Other protective clothing (safety helmets, boots, safety glasses, work gloves) should be worn as required to protect against mechanical injury.

only tuberculosis (see above) and meningococci are likely to present a risk.

- Septicemia is a common terminal event and can be caused by many different organisms (often the patient's own flora), most of which present no hazard. Only cases of meningococcal septicemia or of infection with group A streptococci pose a risk. Life-threatening infections with the latter can result from quite trivial injuries.

Gastrointestinal Organisms. Fecal leakage from bodies is very common. All those handling cadavers should

- wear gloves and impervious disposable aprons;
- take care not to contaminate their instruments or their working environment; and
- wash their hands carefully after procedures and before eating.

Table 39.2 Infections Where Bagging is Essential, and Viewing, Embalming, and Hygienic Preparation* Should Not Be Done

Infection
Anthrax
Plague
Rabies
Smallpox
Viral hemorrhagic fevers
Yellow fever
Transmissible spongiform encephalopathies (e.g., Creutzfeldt-Jakob disease)
Streptococcal disease (group A)
Viral hepatitis (B, C, non-A, non-B)

*bagging = placing the body in a plastic body bag
viewing = allowing the bereaved to see, touch, and spend time with the body prior to disposal
embalming = injecting chemical preservatives into the body to slow the process of decay. Cosmetic enhancement of the appearance of the body may be undertaken to improve the appearance for viewing
hygienic preparation = cleaning and tidying the body so it presents a suitable appearance for viewing (an alternative to embalming)

The bodies of those who have died of diseases such as cholera or typhoid should not be buried in places where they could contaminate water sources.

Transmissible Spongiform Encephalopathies (TSE). The causative agents of these diseases are highly resistant to most disinfectants and to heat. They are not killed by formalin. Exposure to sodium hypochlorite containing 20,000 ppm available chlorine (for at least 1 hour), to 1 to 2M sodium hydroxide, or to steam autoclaving at 134°C for at least 18 minutes is required for decontamination. The skulls of those who have died of CJD or other high-risk infections should only be opened inside a large plastic bag fitted over the head and neck of the cadaver.

Hepatitis.
- Hepatitis A is transmitted by the fecal-oral route and presents the same hazard as other gastrointestinal pathogens. A highly effective vaccine is available.
- Hepatitis B is extremely infectious, and the incidence of this infection continues to increase in many countries. Staff working in hospital mortuaries and embalmers should receive immunization against hepatitis B. The bodies of those who have died of, or were known to be infected with, this virus should be handled only by those wearing full protective clothing.
- Hepatitis C also is infectious, although probably less so than hepatitis B. It is transmitted by the same routes as hepatitis B. There is no vaccine, and similar precautions to those for hepatitis B should be taken.

Human Immunodeficiency Virus. The routes of transmission of hepatitis B and of HIV are similar, and the precautions required to prevent the transmission of HBV should be adequate to prevent transmission of HIV. HIV is probably about 1000-fold less infectious than hepatitis B, and the risk to those handling infected cadavers is therefore proportionately less. Human immunodeficiency virus can survive for many days post mortem in tissues preserved under laboratory conditions. Care should be taken when handling unfixed, HIV-infected material from cadavers, or when undertaking postmortem examinations of those infected with HIV. The embalming of bodies of those known or suspected of being infected is not recommended.

Those infected with HIV are often infected with other organisms (such as mycobacteria), which may be more infectious (albeit less dangerous) than the HIV infection itself.

Viral Hemorrhagic Fevers. Viruses such as Ebola and Marburg are highly infectious and are readily transmitted by contact with infected blood, secretions, and organs. Most of the known outbreaks have been nosocomial. Great care should be exercised when dealing with those who have died of such infections. Staff should wear gloves and protective gowns and masks; postmortem examinations should not be carried out. Bodies should be bagged as soon as possible and should be burned.

Reduction of Risk

Postmortem Rooms.
- Postmortem rooms should be laid out so that the risks to those working in them are minimized. Provision of proper ventilation, running water, and good drainage are all essential.
- Workers should wash their hands after each procedure and before eating (or smoking).
- The environment should be cleaned with a phenolic disinfectant daily.
- Instruments should be washed in a washer-disinfector, autoclaved, or immersed in a phenolic disinfectant for 20 minutes. There are several reasons for the use of a phenolic disinfectant rather than hypochlorite:
  - Hypochlorite is corrosive and may damage surfaces or instruments.
  - Chlorine gas is released when hypochlorite is used and cleaning large areas may lead to unacceptable levels of chlorine in the air.

– Formaldehyde is likely to be present in postmortem rooms (and embalmers' premises) and the reaction between hypochlorite and formaldehyde produces a potent carcinogen, bis(chloromethyl)ether.

Preparation of the Dead for Funerals.

• In many countries, particularly the hotter ones, burial or other disposal of the cadaver follows death within 24 hours (either for practical or religious reasons). Under these circumstances some pathogens may still be viable and appropriate protective clothing and/or good personal hygiene by those handling the deceased is essential.

• Embalming may be undertaken as a means of temporary preservation by reducing microbial activity and slowing decomposition. The embalming of cadavers which have been in accidents or which have been the subjects of postmortem examinations is more difficult. They may be badly damaged and present particular hazards because damaged bones, bone splinters, and occasionally other sharp items, such as needles, are left in the body. Cosmetic work on cadavers may also present hazards if the body has been damaged.

• In most instances only a simple "hygienic preparation" may be carried out, frequently by relatives or religious leaders. This usually involves washing the face and hands, dressing the cadaver, tidying the hair, and possibly trimming the nails and shaving. If there is considered to be a low level of risk, then the use of gloves and simple protective clothing by anyone handling the bodies is an acceptable and effective safety measure.

• In some instances, for example where the person has died of a highly infectious disease such as Ebola or hepatitis B, even hygienic preparation is not safe.

A list of such infections is given in Table 39.2.

• All instruments used for embalming or for preparing bodies for the funeral should be cleaned in hot water and detergent and disinfected, preferably by a brief boil, (five minutes) or by being soaked in a phenolic disinfectant for 20 minutes. Phenolic disinfectants should be used to clean up any spills of blood or body fluid, and single-use gloves should be used to protect the hands from contact with the spill. Hands should always be washed after finishing a session.

Emergency Service Personnel.

- The major hazard facing emergency service personnel is spilled blood. Any risk can be greatly reduced by preventing contact with blood through the use of gloves, face and eye protection, and protective clothing where necessary.

- Bodies that have been decaying for some time, particularly those that have been in water for extended periods of time, present little risk. The organisms likely to be present are their own body flora and water or environmental organisms. The use of proper protective clothing will protect personnel handling such material.

- Bodies should always be transported to mortuary facilities in waterproof body bags or fiberglass temporary coffins.

Disposal of the Dead.

Each society has its own method of disposal of the deceased. These must be respected as far as possible although in a few instances (such as deaths due to highly infectious agents such as Ebola), cremation may be the only safe procedure.

Sometimes, natural or man-made disasters may mean that the normal disposal procedures cannot be followed. Under these circumstances, care must be taken to ensure that the disposal of human remains does not face an already stressed population with further risks. Ideally, bodies should be cremated but if this is not possible, burial with at least one meter/yard of earth over the cadavers (to prevent access by scavengers and pests) is a satisfactory alternative. Religious and social practices should be followed as far as possible. Burial sites must be chosen so as to avoid the risk of water sources being contaminated.

References

Ball J, Desselberger U, Whitwell H. Long-lasting viability of HIV after patient's death. Lancet 1991;338:63.

Gable MR. Hazard: formaldehyde and hypochlorites. Lab Anim 1977;11:61.

Hawkey PM, Pedler SJ, Southall PJ. *Streptococcus pyogenes*: a forgotten occupational hazard in the mortuary. BMJ 1980;281: 1058.

Morris SI. Tuberculosis as an occupational hazard during medical training. Am Rev Tuberculosis 1946;54:140–58.

Newsom SWB, Rowlands C, Mathews J, Elliott CJ. Aerosols in the mortuary. J Clin Pathol 1938;36:137–2.

West DJ. The risk of hepatitis B infection among health professionals in the United States: a review. Am J Med Sci 1984;287:26–33.

Wolff HL, Croon JAB. The survival of smallpox virus (variola minor) in natural circumstances. Bull World Health Organ 1968;38:492–3.

INDEX